THE UNAPOLOGETIC
FAT GIRL'S GUIDE TO EXERCISE
AND OTHER INCENDIARY ACTS

THE
UNAPOLOGETIC
FAT GIRL'S GUIDE
TO EXERCISE
AND OTHER INCENDIARY ACTS

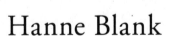

Hanne Blank

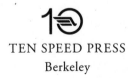

TEN SPEED PRESS

Berkeley

Published in the United States by Ten Speed Press, an imprint of the
Crown Publishing Group, a division of Random House, Inc., New York.
www.crownpublishing.com
www.tenspeed.com

Ten Speed Press and the Ten Speed Press colophon are registered trademarks
of Random House, Inc.

Front cover photograph copyright © 2012 by Substantia Jones of Adipositivity.com
Back cover photograph copyright © Sergey Mironov/Shutterstock.com
Interior photographs, page iii, 10, 46, 70, 102, 130, and 164 copyright © Sergey
Mironov/Shutterstock.com, page 9 copyright © Deymos/Shutterstock.com, page 45
copyright © Lasse Kristensen/Shutterstock.com, page 69 copyright © Kitch Bain/
Shutterstock.com, page 101 copyright © Blazej Lyjak/Shutterstock.com, page 129
copyright © nito/Shutterstock.com, page 163 copyright © 06photo/Shutterstock.com.

Library of Congress Cataloging-in-Publication Data
Blank, Hanne.
  The unapologetic fat girl's guide to exercise and other incendiary acts / Hanne Blank.
    p. cm.
  Includes index.
  Summary: "This empowering exercise guide is big on attitude, giving plus-size women
the motivation, support, and information they need to move their bodies and improve
their health" —Provided by publisher.
  1. Overweight women—Psychology. 2. Overweight women—Health and hygiene.
  3. Exercise for women. 4. Physical fitness for women. I. Title.
  RC522.O25B53 2012
  613.71082—dc23

                        2012023600

ISBN 978-1-60774-286-9
eISBN 978-1-60774-287-6

Printed in the United States of America

Design by Chloe Rawlins

10 9 8 7 6 5 4 3 2 1

First Edition

For Benjamin Lee,
who understands that sometimes,
push-ups are performance art.

Contents

CHAPTER 3

What Am I Going To Do?

CHAPTER 4

Hit the Ground Running

CHAPTER 5

Action and Reaction

CHAPTER 6

Troubleshooting

Acknowledgments

So many people became part of this book, through interviews, conversations, reviewing material as I wrote it, working out with me, supporting me as I developed my own body practice, teaching me, and caring about this book and about fat women's right to joyful and whole-hearted exercise. I thank each and every one of them, from the bottom of my heart. Special thanks are due to Michelle Allison, Linda Bacon, Bear Bergman, Kelly Bliss, Benjamin Lee Buckley, Casey Buss, Leigh Ann Craig, Jeanette DePatie, Malcolm Gin, Abby Lentz, Natalie Luhrs, Keridwen Luis, Jude McLaughlin, Margaret McManus LPN, Michaela Null, Ragen Chastain, Molly Price, Jeannette Smyth, Mary Sykes, Cheryl Wade, Rhetta Wiley, and each and every one of my Warrior Chickens. Additional thanks are due to the gifted and caring professionals at Chase Brexton Health Services, the staff of the 33rd Street Weinberg YMCA, Union Memorial Hospital, and the Welch Medical Library of Johns Hopkins University (all in Baltimore, Maryland), and to Lisa Westmoreland and Christopher Schelling, whose collegial faith and support are the stuff of legend.

Introduction:
Excuse Me—I Think This Is Yours

I want to get one thing straight right from the start: I am not a natural-born jock. I am about as intrinsically athletic as an oyster, with the innate grace and sporty prowess of a brick—a very cute oyster and a very intelligent brick, if I do say so myself, but oysterly and bricklike nevertheless.

Nor do I count a boundless and cheerful appetite for physical activity among my virtues. I will admit that I have grown to appreciate movement and exercise very much, and often now I even enjoy them. But I am bookish and brainy by nature, which, combined with my lack of organic athleticism and physical talents, has made me a lifelong fan of sitting on my abundant and resilient *tuchis*, doing things like, oh, say, writing books. Also I am, quite frankly, not terribly fond of sweating. Much as I might wish it were otherwise, I could count on my fingers the mornings on which I have woken up thinking how much I was looking forward to going on that long brisk walk or that invigorating stint at the gym, and I might not even have to use both hands.

I want to begin this book by telling you this because I need you to know that I am so very not the kind of girl anyone would've voted "Most Likely to Write an Exercise Guide" in the high school yearbook. I am, and have always been, pretty geeky. I live, and have always lived, in my head a lot. I have always been, and most definitely still am, a bit of a klutz. And, although I have been a number of different sizes of fat in my time, I am also a lifelong fat girl.

By this I don't mean pudgy or a little thickwaisted or "someone who could stand to lose a few pounds." I mean actually, honest-to-God, Lane Bryant-shoppin', belly-and-butt-shots-on-the-TV-news-resemblin', nasty-comments-from-random-strangers-gettin', fat. In my adult life, I have never weighed less than two hundred pounds. I have often weighed quite a lot more. The phrase "morbidly obese" was first used about me, in my presence, when I was still in grammar school, and despite the frequency with which I have been described—if you'll excuse my translating the phrase slightly inaccurately—as "sick fat," I continue existing, healthily, and fatly.

I also exercise a lot. You heard me right. I exercise. Frequently. Five or six days a week, most weeks. Sometimes seven. Once a day. Or sometimes twice. Occasionally three times, but I reserve that sort of silliness for weekends and vacations, because who has time to go swimming *and* for a nice long walk *and* ride bikes during the workweek? Sometimes I exercise energetically, sometimes lackadaisically, sometimes joyously, sometimes meditatively, and sometimes with a virtuosic and well-honed grumpiness that puts even my eighteen-year-old cat to shame. (Some days I manage all of these emotional states in a single gym session. It's very *The Many Moods of Me Moving My Big Ol' Carcass* around here sometimes.)

The point is, I exercise—not, as I think I have made pretty clear, because I'm one of those folks who by gosh, just *lives* to exercise. Nor do I think that exercising makes me or anyone any sort of model citizen or moral paragon: to me morality has more to do with how one treats *other people*. I exercise because I think it's important. Rather, I *know* it's important.

It may be that exercise is somewhat more important for me than it might be for some other people. My particular body has a very specific and dramatic relationship to exercise. For me, finding out firsthand just how profoundly regular exercise affected my body's ability to use its own insulin convinced me that exercise was more than just Something You're Supposed to Do; it was quite literally powerful medicine. Also there are a number of other ways that exercising regularly improves my physical and mental health. And I have noticed that this seems to be true for many other people as well. It's been very illuminating to observe what happens for friends and loved ones when they do and don't exercise regularly: the seasonal depression that responds as much to walking to work as it does to the big expensive full-spectrum light box, the angina that only acts up when someone's been too busy to get to karate class, the edema in the legs that gets so much better after a trip to the pool. It doesn't seem to matter what size someone is. The beneficial side effects movement has on the body's ability to maintain a healthy physical equilibrium appear to be among the few things in this world that seem genuinely to be one-size-fits-all.

But the whole "exercise is good for your health" thing isn't what I find most important about exercise. It's not even the most compelling, in the long run. Exercise, after all, doesn't make you immortal or even bulletproof. There are plenty of health conditions that exercise can't and won't change. You have no idea how much I wish exercise could rid me of my allergy to dairy products, for example, but I could run and lift weights and do sit-ups from sunup to sundown and the math would still look like me + mac and cheese = Technicolor Yawn. Nor does exercise permanently solve my body's ongoing and entrenched tendency to refuse to use its own perfectly good insulin. If I stop exercising regularly, my body turns up its metabolic nose like a thirteen-year-old girl with a grudge at the insulin it produces.

Exercise is not a panacea and it is not a magic wand. There are lots of ways our bodies can break that exercise can't fix. There are lots of ways our bodies can be dysfunctional that exercise can't even help. Human beings are fragile and complicated, and how or whether we move ourselves around is just one part of the picture. And yet, it is my considered stance that exercise is crucially important. Even if you're fat. No, strike that—what I should've said is that exercise is crucially important, *especially* if you're fat.

Exercise is not important because it'll make you thin (it won't necessarily do anything of the kind) or because it'll give you perfect and enduring health (it won't necessarily do that either). But, as I discovered more or less by accident in the course of exercising as medical therapy, exercise does something else that is, in its way, more remarkable. Exercise—by which I mean regular physical movement that puts your body through its paces—is crucially important because it is something that makes it possible for you and your body to coexist in better and more integrated ways. It builds a bridge across the mind-body split. Moving your body, regularly and with intent, makes you secure in your own body in a way that no amount of above-the-neck effort can duplicate. Being secure in your body, my friends, is a thing that is relevant to the interests of pretty much every fat girl I have ever known (and a great many other people, too).

I know, I know: right now, some of you may be thinking I sound a little deranged. You may be wondering if I've been sucked into some nutty elliptical trainer cult or something. Believe me when I say that sometimes these kinds of sentiments come out of my mouth, and I give myself the "who are you and what have you done with Hanne?" stinkeye. I never expected to find myself an exercise evangelist. Hell, I never expected to find myself being even so much as an exercise apologist. But then again, I never expected to find myself experiencing exercise as a source of genuine well-being or amazement or find myself having exercise-induced epiphanies. And I definitely never expected to find that I was the kind of person for whom exercising was an indispensable part of feeling like I was genuinely the best and most fully present version of myself.

I know it sounds weird. I know it sounds wifty and new-agey and like a big crock of bong water. I mean, I'm a fat girl, you know? I've been that way all my life. As my fellow lifelong fat girls are well aware, we have to keep a calm head when it comes to people yammering on at us about how great exercising is, because we know full well it's almost always code for "Hey fatass, if you broke a sweat now and then it might help with the lard factor." This makes us skeptical on the topic, at the very least. Heaven knows that even after many years of regular gym-rattitude, I *still* automatically snarl like a rabid Rottweiler whenever someone comes at me with the whole bright-eyed, bushy-tailed, I'm-going-to-lead-the-fat-girl-to-the-light routine about the glories and wonders of exercise.

Yet here I am, trying to get you to take me seriously about the glories and wonders of exercise.

I'm not doing it because I care whether you lose weight or not. I'm not doing it to play the "concern for your health" card that is so often really just a veiled "I want you to lose weight" thing. I'm not even doing it because I think there's a chance that exercise might improve your actual real bodily and mental health, even though there is a pretty good chance that it will. I'm trying to talk you into taking me seriously about exercise because there's more to this exercise thing than you think. There has to be. If even I, with my natural (and, I still maintain, entirely defensible) disinclination toward anything that makes me sweaty without offering at least the balancing prospect of orgasms, have invested my time and energy and love into making exercise a near-daily part of my life, there has to be something real, something genuine, something way beyond the superficial or the obvious that has its hooks into me.

That thing is this: exercise gives your body to you. It blows the dust off and it gives it a little shine and it hands it over with a weird little curtsey that makes you understand, maybe for the first time, that this body of yours is actually kind of wonderful, maybe even miraculous. Movement teaches you, in visceral, wordless ways similar to the ways that sex does, what your body is all about. Most of all, it teaches you that your body is not just a sort of jar made out of meat that you lug around because it's what you keep your brain in, but an equal and in fact quite opinionated and demonstrative partner in the joint production that is you. Exercise keeps you honest about this. When you forget, it taps you on the shoulder, points to your body, and says "Excuse me, I believe this is yours."

It can be unsettling and strange to have this happen. Many of us, particularly those of us who are fat, spend a lot of time living *with* our bodies but not really *in* them. You can't really blame us; the culture we live in is so hateful and abusive toward everybody and every body that doesn't measure up to its constantly shifting targets for "perfect" that it can be really painful and unpleasant to spend too much time really fully inhabiting your inevitably imperfect body. When exercise brings you back to your body, it can be very unfamiliar, uncomfortable, and scary, particularly when your body still isn't "perfect" (whatever *that* is). It is not much fun being fully in your body when you're sort of a stranger there, and it is definitely not fun being in your body when you are constantly cringing and waiting for the next slap or slur or nasty, snarling laugh.

Fortunately, exercise helps with all this. It makes you stronger, not just in the sense that your body gets more sturdy and skilled. Your mind gets stronger, too. The same exercise that says "Excuse me, I believe this is yours" is building bridges between your body and your brain. As you get more physically fluent, you also get stronger in the sense of being more at home and secure in yourself, more effortlessly confident, more organically sure that your body is a good place to be—dependable and capable and worthwhile. The slaps and slurs and laughs may still happen sometimes (another thing exercise can't cure is the fact that other people's children can be massive assholes). But you've gotten stronger, too strong and too focused to give a damn about something so inconsequential as a stranger's unsolicited opinion. "Get out of my way," you snap as you walk smartly past. "I've got *things to do*."

Because, ya know, you do, and not easy things, either. Exercising is complicated and hard, especially when you've got Body Issues and maybe Fitness Issues and also Gym-Clothes Problems and probably Fat-Kid-in-Gym-Class issues and Holy-Crap-Locker-Room-History Issues and all that *stuff* to navigate. And just like I won't lie and tell you that exercise is all about health or all about weight or size or "body sculpting" or how many miles you can run before you puke up your socks, I won't blow smoke up your ass about how exercise is so easy either. (Besides, you'd know I was lying. As I've said to other people many times, fat does not equal stupid.)

If exercise were easy, if moving your body regularly and freely and well were simple, there'd be no need for this book. If listening to your body and giving it the weird inconvenient things it asks for were complete child's play, you'd already be doing it. If carving out time to do something that maybe feels stupid and embarrassing (but also really important and revelatory) were something people did nonchalantly and without having to think about it, well, you just *would*. If getting the exercise that lets you be completely at home in your body were really as simple as a pair of Nikes and a no-nonsense "just do it" approach, you wouldn't have to stand there in the bookstore holding this book, trying to decide whether you're really ready (because reading it might change things, and change is scary) to actually buy it and take it home and read the rest of it—to say nothing of actually making some additions or changes to the ways you use and move this wonderful body of yours.

This stuff isn't easy. That's why I wrote this book. Because, um, excuse me, this body you're in? Yeah, I think that's yours. You're the only one who can provide it with the things that help it work better and feel better, and help *you* work better and feel better and think better with regard to your body and your self. (And yes, I am totally right there with you in thinking that it would be a whole lot more palatable if you could get the same results from caffeine, chocolate, and Internet Scrabble.) It's not necessarily convenient. It's not necessarily fun. But it's worth doing and it can be done, especially with a little help from someone who's been there and gets it.

Moving your body—it's a thing. And it's worth it because you are, too.

And with that, here's a disclaimer: This book is not a replacement for medical treatment or in-person fitness instruction. Every effort has been made to make the information given in this book accurate and practical. Inevitably, not all fitness or health advice is appropriate for all people or all situations. I hope that you do, in fact, try this at home. But if you do, understand that you do it at your own risk.

INCENDIARY ACT #1

REFUSE TO APOLOGIZE FOR HAVING A BODY

You never have to apologize for having a body—never, not once. Without your body, you wouldn't be here at all. It is the prerequisite for absolutely everything you have ever done and everything you will ever do, everything you have ever been and everything you might be someday. In order to be, you must have a body. Call it an accident of birth.

That's why you don't have to apologize for it: because apologizing for having a body is basically the same thing as apologizing for being alive. And being alive is something for which no one ever needs to apologize. As the brilliant and fat performer Glenn Marla so memorably puts it: *there is no wrong way to have a body.*

So don't apologize for your body. Live in it!

You only have the one body, you know, and it's a limited-time offer. So you might as well enjoy it while you've got it.

Even when you're not actively enjoying your body—and we all have those moments and those days—respect it. Honor its right to exist. You don't have to love absolutely everything about your body all the time. But you can always recognize that your body, in this moment, has the right to exist just as it is.

One of my favorite Gay Pride parade marching chants has always been "We're here! We're queer! We're fabulous! Get used to it!" It's a sentiment that translates just as well to having a body. We're here! We have bodies! They're fabulous! Get used to it!

CHAPTER 1

Why Bother?

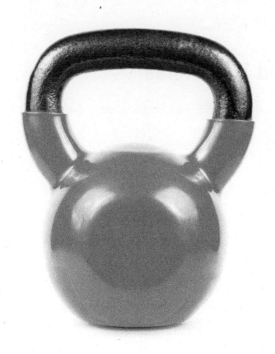

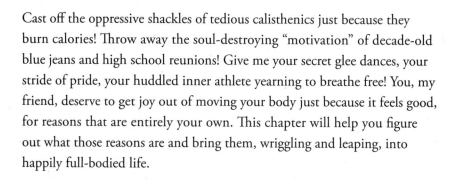

Cast off the oppressive shackles of tedious calisthenics just because they burn calories! Throw away the soul-destroying "motivation" of decade-old blue jeans and high school reunions! Give me your secret glee dances, your stride of pride, your huddled inner athlete yearning to breathe free! You, my friend, deserve to get joy out of moving your body just because it feels good, for reasons that are entirely your own. This chapter will help you figure out what those reasons are and bring them, wriggling and leaping, into happily full-bodied life.

Whys and Wherefores

People pick up books about exercise for a lot of different reasons. Doubtless you've got your own reasons . . . perhaps more than one.

- Maybe you're looking for a change, or a challenge, and think that taking up a new physical activity sounds interesting but you need some encouragement.

- Maybe you're an athlete whose body has changed and you're finding it hard to get back in the game in a body that doesn't look or feel—and may also not work—the way you remember.

- Maybe you're hoping that this will be the book that finally does the trick and you'll become thin. (Fair warning: This may very well not be what happens. And that's okay. It's only a book, after all, not a magic wand.)

- Maybe you've been given an "Exercise or else!" ultimatum by your doctor and you're clutching desperately at anything that seems like it'll help . . . or at least get your doctor off your back.

- Maybe you've always been kind of interested in sports or exercise but hate feeling like everyone thinks you'll never be able to do it or that you have no right to try because you're fat.

- Or maybe you've been interested in exercising more for a while but really resent the assumption that the only reason any fat person would do that is weight loss.

- Maybe you are hopeful that if you can figure out how to move your body more and make it stick, you'll feel better and have more energy.

- Maybe you have a specific medical issue that you'd like to try to improve through more and better movement.

- Maybe you've been trying to exercise more but fat-related issues have you feeling stuck, or stymied, or scared: What if you're the only fat woman in the locker room? Or you're scared you'll burst the Swiss ball, break the elliptical trainer, or not be able to get up off the yoga class floor once you get down there? What if you have major PTSD from being humiliated by gym teachers? Or you don't know where to find a swimsuit or a sports bra or for that matter a bicycle that can take everything you've got?

Or maybe your reason is none of these things. Maybe it's something else entirely, something you can't quite articulate. Maybe you're just one of the many, many people who has a vague, nagging, guilty sense that you should exercise more even though you don't really want to and you're not sure you see the point.

Whatever your reason for picking up this book or for looking into increasing the amount of movement in your life, I hope that I can convince you to entertain one more possibility: you should consider moving your body more just because it's your birthright. That's right, it is your God-given right to have the freedom, the ability, and the confidence to move your body freely and happily in the world. Creating and maintaining a body practice that includes movement and exertion that you enjoy, that gives you strength and flexibility and skills, helps make that happen.

This is one of the reasons this book is entitled *The Unapologetic Fat Girl's Guide to Exercise and Other Incendiary Acts*. Our culture often expects women in general, and fat women in particular, to confine and limit themselves. We are often discouraged, in many different ways, from moving freely, playfully, and happily in the world. We're not supposed to take up space and be visible and spontaneous and dynamic, colorful or loud or boisterous or rambunctious. Heaven knows we're not supposed to be fierce, physically unafraid, and fully aware of our own physical power. To which I say: screw that.

All these are reasons why moving your body, and particularly moving your fat body, can truly be an incendiary act. When we move our bodies for the sake of our own enjoyment and well-being, not because we're trying to look a certain way or as a way of paying for the "sin" of being fat, it's a pretty serious form of rebellion.

When we exercise because we like being strong and flexible and we like having the kind of stamina and power it takes to change the world (rather than because we're "bad" or "undisciplined" or we're "lazy" or "let ourselves go"), it's a way of thumbing our noses at all the people who've ever tried to tell us that we or our bodies were unworthy.

When our body practice includes the kinds of movement that help us improve our mental and physical functioning, it's a way of taking things into our own hands in terms of our health and our experience of our bodies.

When we move around freely in the world in our bodies of all different shapes and sizes and colors and abilities and talents, we prove to ourselves and to other people that there are many different ways to happily, actively *be*, to move, to climb and walk and swim and roll and jump and engage with the world and everything in it.

Moving your body helps you do more of the things you want to do, helps you experience and enjoy more of life, and helps you be the expert on and the boss of yourself. Moving your body for your own reasons helps you set your own agendas and give the ones you don't like that were imposed on you without your consent a solid boot to the head. The fact that it often helps you be healthier and recover more quickly when you do get sick is the icing on the cake.

You surely have your own reasons for picking up this book. You surely have your own reasons for wanting to exercise. But now you have one more: because it's an incendiary act. It can change your life and it can change the world.

A Note on the F-Word

Throughout this book, I happily and freely drop the F-bomb—no, not the famous four-letter word that rhymes with duck. It's the other one. You know: *fat*.

I know that a lot of you reading this will cringe the first few times you see it, maybe even the first few dozen times. But you'll get used to it. It'll become just another word that can be used to describe bodies, like short or bald or lanky or freckled.

That's the point. "Fat" is, you know, just another word that can be used to describe bodies. Fat bodies are bodies just like any other bodies. They deserve the same respect, the same nurture, the same care, and the same attention as any other.

There's also another side to this, namely, self-defense. If you can learn to read, hear, and use the word "fat" as a normal word, an everyday word, a word you can use to describe things without flinching or apologizing, it generally stops being a weapon other people can use to hurt you. By making the word your own, by using it appropriately and without rancor, you make it yours.

Part of the reason I wrote this book was to help you find ways to be happier, more comfortable, and healthier in your own body and your relationship with your body. Moving your body with as much respect and joy as you can possibly muster is an absolutely critical part of this. And so is being able to talk about, and hear about, your own body with the same kind of respect and joy, happiness, comfort, and health.

So, yeah. Fat. Fat, fat, fat! Say it a few dozen times until it sounds silly when you say it.

I'm fat. You might be fat too. Fat, my dear reader, isn't something we're going to let stop us from grabbing life by the ears or from hitting the gym, the pool, the trail, the street, or anywhere else we happen to want to leap and run, swim and bike, stride and strut, as fat and sassy as we please, to our fat little hearts' content.

30 THINGS TO LOVE ABOUT EXERCISE

(None of Which Have Anything to Do with Your Weight, Your Size, or What You Look Like)

1. Working out is an immune-system booster, which is great since no one actually enjoys being a mobile snot fountain.

2. Exercise builds ferociously sturdy little old ladies (and men): it's fantastic for your bones, reduces the risk of Alzheimer's, and improves balance and coordination.

3. Exercise reduces symptoms of both depression and anxiety. Organic, legal DIY mellowness is a pretty sweet side effect.

4. Working out helps regulate your blood pressure, reducing the effects of things like traffic jams and not being allowed to strangle that one coworker who really, really needs it.

5. Exercising makes you smarter: research shows that exercise incorporating complex movement, especially, makes people learn better and faster.

6. Working out hath charms to soothe the savage metabolic system, encouraging insulin sensitivity and making diabetes management a little easier.

7. Regular exercise tends to generate major mojo. And by mojo, I mean increased sex drive and sexual responsivity. Yeah, baby.

8. If you suffer from insomnia, exercise helps, and not just because it tires you out; it also helps your body regulate its own rhythms.

9. Workouts boost levels of neurochemicals like dopamine and serotonin, which is like getting a biochemical massage in terms of counteracting stress.

10. You'll be able to sing louder and dive deeper with your improved lung capacity.

11. Your joints get stronger and less prone to injuries and diseases, including tricky ones like repetitive stress injuries and arthritis.

12. It enables you to satisfy those urges to reenact dance numbers from Broadway musicals. So what if you're in the grocery store?

13. Will you be able to snatch a speeding bullet out of the air? Maybe not, but working out does improve people's reaction time.

14. Endorphins—mmmmm, sweet, sweet endorphins: the "runner's high" isn't just for runners, ya know.

15. Outrunning the zombies.

16. It makes you strong. You never know when you'll need to be that person who can carry the suitcase full of gold bars through the airport without anyone being able to tell that it's so heavy.

17. Your body and your brain get superbly and thoroughly oxygenated, which tends to make you feel peppy and full of mischief.

18. Most of us like to think we're flexible people who can roll with the punches. Exercising makes it more likely that it'll literally be true, not just figuratively.

19. If, God forbid, you should get sick, being a regular exerciser can help reduce the length and severity of your illness. It has even been shown to reduce cancer mortality for some kinds of cancer.

20. Exercise can help pregnancy and labor go a lot more smoothly. Afterward, it helps you keep up with the kid.

21. Probiotics and antacids have their place, but if you want to give your digestive system the best possible advantage, there's nothing like fiber, water, and exercise.

continued

22. Physical competence—just knowing you can count on your body to do stuff effectively and without trouble—is pretty damn nice.

23. It makes your heart happy and efficient to the point that your resting heart rate may get lower.

24. Four words: Exercise-induced mitochondrial biogenesis—exercising can increase the number of mitochondria in your muscle cells, which is just completely geeky cool.

25. Stamina: "Another ten rounds? Sure," you say. "Bring it . . . *if you can.*"

26. You're much less likely to fall and much more likely to be able to get right back up and brush yourself off if you do.

27. It's kind of nice not to think twice about getting down on the floor to look for that thing that just rolled under the entertainment center or about how you'll get up again.

28. It's eco-friendly. No matter how much you sweat or how hard you breathe, you will not produce toxic waste or greenhouse gases.

29. It gives you a bulletproof excuse. "Sorry, Aunt Linda, of course I'd love to hear all about your colonoscopy, but I have to go or I'll be late to Pilates."

30. Juicy ideas and spicy epiphanies seem to be attracted to sweat and gym socks. Moving your body is a fantastic way to jump-start your brain.

What Do You Think You're Doing?

It's useful to know what you think you're doing when you move your body. We don't move our bodies in a vacuum. Even if we are all alone, each of us still has our own relationship with our body, and our own history with our body and with movement, to contend with. We carry around a lot of emotions, ideas, and memories, and they can exert powerful influence. The more we know about what we think we're doing when we move our bodies, the more we can work with ourselves to make our movement more satisfying and sustainable.

Getting a clear picture of what those thoughts are can be hard. When they are all inside, swirling around your head, it can be easy not to recognize your own thoughts or admit that they're there. Without some sort of reality check, and some sort of outside perspective, it can be hard to recognize that your thoughts are just that—your thoughts—and not some sort of magical universal truths about movement. (It's a pretty good bet they're not.)

To help yourself get some perspective on what's going on in your own head with regard to physical activity, take a few minutes with a pen and paper, your journal, or something along those lines, and see if you can answer these questions:

1. What do you imagine happens to your body when you are physically active? How does your body behave and feel different when you're moving?

2. How would you like moving your body to make you feel?

3. What one thing do you wish everyone understood about what physical activity is like for you?

4. What's your biggest fear with regard to physical activity? What things are you most worried about in relation to moving your body more?

5. What's your biggest fantasy with regard to physical activity? What do you dream of when you think about adding more movement to your life?

6. What things are you most excited about in relation to moving your body?

Read through your answers and see what you have to say. When you see them all written out, what pictures emerge?

Questions 1 and 2 should help you think about what you think you're doing in terms of ideals and goals. They should specifically tell you a few things about what you want to, or think you should, *feel* with regard to movement. That's important because how you feel will actually play a bigger role in making sure you continue to pursue physical activity than anything else. It's very hard to keep challenging yourself to do difficult things if you don't feel that, subjectively, you're having a positive experience. This doesn't mean that it has to be some wild extravaganza of unbridled bliss (but hey, if you can make that happen, go for it!). But it does mean you want to get something good out of it. You want to feel like you're doing something right. The answers to these questions will tell you what some of those things are for you right now and give you something to work for and look for.

Questions 3 and 4 are about what you think you're doing in terms of your psychological boundaries. These questions will tell you something about what kinds of experiences are really emotionally important to you, what things frighten you, and what things are likely to make you unhappy or uncomfortable. These are important because when we have too many experiences that are painful or unhappy, or the things that are deeply emotionally important to us get ignored, we're likely to avoid those situations. You want to have every advantage when it comes to creating an environment in your life where you can move your body happily or at least neutrally. Knowing where these hot buttons are for you will help you work around them and also help you recognize that when those buttons get pushed, you're upset for a reason . . . and it's not the end of the world—it's just that your buttons got pushed.

Questions 5 and 6 are about what you think you're doing in terms of motivation. Your answers to these questions tell you what makes you want to do what you're doing, what you can count on to help you feel excited and eager, and where your best rewards are going to come from. When you're doing something physically and emotionally challenging like adding more physical movement to your life, it's good to have specific, tangible reminders of what's in it for you. It's also really good to remind yourself of the good things when they happen. Having it in writing helps you stay aware and conscious of these things.

Body Practice

They say that practice makes perfect, but that isn't quite true. What practice really does is make you competent, then refines your skill into fluency. Whether you're learning to play piano, perform a role in a play, change a diaper, bake a loaf of bread, or most anything else, it's the same basic story. You start out awkward and halting, but repetition makes things smoother until eventually you know what you're doing: you don't have to try too hard or think about it too much. This is when, to people watching you, you make it look easy.

Exactly the same thing is true about living fully in your body and taking advantage of your innate physical capacities for movement and activity. Being comfortable moving around and being active, and feeling like it's something you can be good at, takes practice.

Modern life doesn't engage our bodies very fully much of the time. Our jobs are often pretty sedentary. We spend a lot of time in our cars or taking various forms of motorized transit. Our daily routines are often repetitive and limited. The kinds of recreational things we enjoy are often largely passive, from a physical point of view. Many of us don't, in short, spend a lot of time practicing the art and craft of living fully in our bodies or practicing a range of the many physical things that our bodies can do. That's our cultural baseline, and it's kind of a shame. Our bodies are wonderful things, capable of so much that is fabulous and fun, and yet so often we don't give them much chance to shine.

Being fat may mean, for some of us, that we engage with our bodies even less. It's easy to understand why. Fatness is heavily stigmatized. Many people simply assume that fat people are incapable of a rich, interesting physical existence. Even more insidiously, there's a common belief that fat people don't *deserve* to have good active relationships with their physical bodies. People may think fat bodies are too unsightly to be seen moving around or wearing exercise clothes, that these are privileges that only thin people with "good" and conventionally attractive bodies should enjoy. We might believe these things ourselves. After all, we're hardly immune to the messages society teaches just because we're getting the short end of the stick. Even if we aren't very fat—or not fat at all—self-judgment and the fear of others' judgment may be enough to convince us to keep ourselves from being as active and as participatory as we'd like to be.

Adding to this, most of us learn as early as the kindergarten playground or grade school gym class that when we are active and move our fat bodies, it can make us targets for all kinds of cruel, condescending, and mean-spirited treatment. There's nothing innate about fat bodies that prevents us from having good relationships with them. There's nothing inherent to fatness that keeps fat people from being as active and as dynamic as anybody else. But there are a lot of attitudes and prejudices that can easily turn "Fat people don't exercise" into a self-fulfilling prophecy.

This can be hard to get past. No matter how much we like the idea of being more active, if you're fat—even just a little—you probably have a lifetime of crappy anti-fat bias and negativity to grapple with. Getting in the game and actually *being* active, when you're fat, can sound like about as much fun as a root canal.

This is the other place that the idea of practice comes into play: practicing moving your body means practicing being a person moving her body in the world (you know, the place where they keep all those other people). Practicing being a person moving her body in the world means practicing being someone who prioritizes putting her energy into moving her body happily and in satisfying ways, not wasting her time and energy on unhelpful, unproductive crap that's just trying to keep her "in her place." Your place is wherever you want it to be, doing whatever kinds of things make you and your body happy. Living that truth takes practice.

And that is the source of my phrase "body practice." Because living fully in your body does take practice. Things won't always go smoothly when you move your body, either physically or socially. Practice is, by nature, something you do regularly, usually something you do every day. Especially at first, you will probably be hypersensitive to what doesn't feel good. You'll feel self-conscious and you'll be hyperaware of everything that seems awkward or clunky or bad.

Practice is what helps you feel less awkward, less clunky, and better. Gradually it makes you faster and stronger and gives you expertise. It doesn't happen all at once, and indeed it may never feel like you reach the end of the road. That's only to be expected. Practice is not something one is ever finished with—it is a practice! But practice does eventually make things that once felt very hard feel easy, and maybe even effortless.

The same is true for the social side of moving your body. The pressure of all that looming potential judgment can be intense. But if there's one thing I have learned in my years of reading women's magazines on the elliptical trainer, as well as talking to friends and family of all sizes and weights, it is that fat women aren't the only ones who experience huge anxiety about what other people may think of their bodies in physical activity contexts. Many women with bodies that are considered "thin" and "fit" and "shapely" experience major body-image freak-outs when they're in group exercise class, working with personal trainers, or simply thinking about buying a swimsuit. Why do you think advertisers make so many millions on the idea that people need to go on diets and exercise themselves to a frazzle before they can let themselves go to the beach? It's not because only fat people are vulnerable to body insecurity, that's for damn sure.

So, when fears or freak-outs get the better of you, take a deep breath and know that you're so very not alone. Putting your fear on the back burner and existing fully and with real presence in your body in spite of it isn't easy, but it gets easier with practice. Body practice helps you feel less vulnerable, less fragile, and better able to deal with it on those occasions when someone decides to be a jerk. Practice makes you strong. It teaches you that yes, my glorious plumpling, you do belong on that gym floor or pool deck or basketball court just like everyone else. Practice means that by and by it gets easy to just look the jerks in the eye and say, "Get out of my way, jerk. I'm late for practice," because you've *practiced*, you've *trained*. And you've gotten *good* at being you, living fully and freely in that fabulous body of yours, and knowing exactly what you want to do with yourself.

What Do You Want to Do with Yourself?

A lot of people set out to add more physical activity to their lives without any sense of why they're doing it aside from a guilty sense of obligation. This guilt is perfectly normal in our culture, of course, but it's far from optimal. Guilt tends to grind away at your sense of well-being, plus it'll lead to resentment over the long haul. Who needs to feel guilty all the time? How depressing!

Much more positive, useful, and way more motivating is to tease out some of the deeper and more specific reasons you're doing what you're doing, and what you *want* to be doing, when you're moving your body.

There are lots of things you might want to learn, improve, have more fun with, be better at, or change your relationship to in the realm of movement and body practice. You might secretly want to learn to do an art or activity that's always appealed to you—aikido or juggling or tango—that you've just never carved out the time to learn. You might want to improve your posture, stamina, balance, reflexes, flexibility, breathing, alignment, or range of motion. You might want to get better at pacing yourself. You might want to get better at the breaststroke or backhand returns, your bench-press form or your free throws. You might want to have more fun being outdoors or in the water or playing with your kids or your dog or going out dancing. You might just want to have more fun because you're more able to be physical in whatever ways crop up. You might want to change your relationship to going to the gym or the pool or to be less scared of being seen moving your body in public. You might want to write yourself some new history with regard to being physically competitive with others, being in a locker room, participating in group exercise, or a million other things.

If you're having trouble thinking of things you want to do with your body practice off the top of your head, try this: Set a timer for ten minutes and sit down with a pen and a piece of paper. Ask yourself, "Okay, self, we're making some changes to our body practice and we're adding more movement: what do you want to get out of it?" Write down whatever comes to mind. It doesn't matter how small or mundane it seems. "I want to be flexible enough that I can pick up a paper clip when I drop one without having it be a big production" is totally legit! It doesn't matter how weird it seems or whether it only really makes sense to you. It doesn't even matter if it's about exorcising demons. Wanting to show your eighth-grade gym teacher how wrong she was about fat girls, just for the record, is a 100-percent-legitimate thing to put on this list. (It's been on mine for a decade, and for the record, Miss Batts, you can kiss my firm-but-pliant ass.)

At the end of ten minutes, take a look at that list. What came up for you when you brainstormed? It might be that you have a lot of things on your list that relate to learning particular skills. You might have a bunch of items that all relate to improving particular aspects of strength and overall condition. Maybe you have a batch of skills you want to hone relating to some kind of activity you already engage in. Maybe it's a mix.

Circle the items on your list that really seem like priorities to you now that you look at them. These will give you some touchstones, some ideas to return to when you need motivation or inspiration, and some things you could specifically arrange to get feedback on so you can know how you are progressing. Write your short list down somewhere that you will remember to look at it from time to time. I have been known to write mine on a sticky note and tuck it into my date book a few months down the line so I will reencounter it automatically when the time comes.

There is one thing you should be wary of when you are figuring out what you want to do with yourself—a particular category of items that might appear on your list that you should approach with extreme caution. These are desires to change the appearance of your body in specific ways. Whether it's "I want to have a flat stomach" or "I want to have big biceps," "I want to be five sizes smaller" or "I want swimmers' shoulders" or whatever it happens to be, these kinds of desires are dangerous simply because they're not things you can necessarily control no matter how much you exercise. If you make the outward appearance or dimensions of your body into your criteria for success, you are more often than not setting yourself up for frustration.

There's a world of difference between "I want to have great upper-body strength" and "I want to have big, super-cut biceps": a person who has great upper-body strength may never have noticeably big or well-defined biceps; her body may not be inclined to grow them that way. Similarly, while you can easily work toward a goal like "improve my core strength and strengthen abdominal muscles," your body may never cooperate with the desire to have a flat stomach even if your weight or amount of body fat changes. For better or worse, our aesthetics cannot alter our genetics. And that's okay. Looking like what you look like is not just okay—it's distinctive and unique and wonderful.

It is easy to fall into the trap of deciding that what you want to do with yourself is to radically change the appearance of your body. But trying to force your body to change is a very good way to frustrate yourself. In the long term, the body's stubborn resistance to magically transform itself into something it has never been (and is not inclined to be) is something that results in a lot of people abandoning exercise with the snarl, "It didn't *do anything*." This is a waste and a shame.

Moving your body does an enormous amount, whether or not your appearance changes in any way at all as a result. For one thing, *it moves your body*. Identifying the things that you want for yourself and your body practice that don't focus on changing your body will help you take good care of your body and give it what it needs to be the best, strongest, sturdiest, most flexible, most resilient, most activity-ready body it can be . . . and that's something that looks good on everybody.

---

25 SAMPLE GOALS FOR YOUR BODY PRACTICE

What goals have you set your sights on for your body practice? Thinking big about things like completing a triathlon or climbing Half Dome might be motivating over the long term. But sometimes big goals just aren't realistic, and in any event, they can be a long, long way off. Postponing any sense of achievement so far into the future that you can't see it from here even if you squint is no fun.

The answer is to find a variety of big and small goals that let you have regular doses of victory along the way. Some should be experiments, where there is no yardstick save your own improvement. For others, a tangible goal—like a distance or a length of time for which you do an exercise—is great. This list of goals offers options for people at many different levels of strength, ability, and stamina. Some can be used by anyone, no matter where they're starting out.

1. Use a pedometer to track your average daily movement for a week. Then, each day for the following week, see if you can hit that earlier average number of steps plus five hundred more.

2. Climb a flight of stairs while carrying on an animated conversation, without breathing hard.

---

3. Learn a new stretch or yoga pose and practice it until you can hold the pose for one minute.

4. Time yourself while you walk a mile at a comfortable pace. Then give yourself one month to work up to doing it two minutes faster but still having it feel just as comfortable.

5. Choose an exercise video and give yourself one month to work up to being able to do the entire thing from beginning to end.

6. Try the Two-Week Variety Challenge: a different physical activity for half an hour a day, every day for two weeks— a great way to try new things and see what you like!

7. Learn three upper-body strength exercises and do them three times a week for a month.

8. Sign up for a 5K. You don't have to run; you can walk, wheel, or push a stroller. . . .

9. Try the One Hundred Sit-Ups or One Hundred Push-Ups challenges. Download the workout plans online. (See the Resource Guide.)

10. Swim five laps without stopping. Master that kick-flip turn to make it all work.

11. Bike your favorite route, but shift the gears up a notch higher than usual. See how long it takes for this to become your new normal.

12. Learn two stretches you can do at regular intervals during the day, and mark off on your calendar whenever you do them. See how long a stretch of unbroken days of stretching you can get on your calendar. When you get to one hundred days, give yourself a prize. (May I suggest a copy of Bob Anderson's classic book, *Stretching*? See the Resource Guide.)

13. Look at trail maps for a nearby state or national park. Pick a trail of reasonable length that you'd really like to hike, call some friends, and pack a fantastic picnic!

continued

14. Sign up for a fitness class of a type you've always wanted to try and finish the series of classes even if the learning curve is steep.

15. Sign up for a charity walk. Raising money for a good cause and increasing your activity level at the same time is a great combination.

16. Pick an errand you do regularly and walk or bike to and from it instead of driving or using public transit.

17. See how many flights of stairs you can climb in a day just going about your usual business.

18. For a month, commit to not letting more than one day go by without some sort of physical activity. If you didn't move your body yesterday, move it today.

19. Just for today, get up and walk around when you're on the phone.

20. Buy or build yourself a treadmill desk so that you can walk very slowly all day while you work.

21. By the end of next month, add five pounds to your weights for all your upper-body weight training.

22. Get together with friends and rent a neighborhood pool for a private swim party to celebrate an upcoming milestone.

23. Have a wedding to attend? Sign up for dance lessons so you can be ready to rock it on the dance floor by the time the day arrives.

24. During the next year, pledge to attend fifty classes of your favorite group exercise class. Celebrate the fiftieth by going out with friends after class.

25. Plan a vacation that includes sightseeing or touring on foot, bike, ski, canoe, or otherwise under your own steam. Train up so you can enjoy that vacation to the fullest!

What Do You Call It?

"Exercise" can sound mighty grim. It brings to mind military maneuvers, legal documents, and being forced to practice the most boring things ever on the piano. It sounds like repetitive, dull, pointless toil of the sort that gives a self-righteous hard-on to the kind of people who are deeply devoted to holier-than-thou smugness.

"Exercise" sounds like what your doctor wants you to do (or your gym teacher or that coworker who is always giving you a hard time about your weight).

"Exercise" sounds like something that you aren't going to like, not like something you'd do for fun. It sounds like something that isn't interesting; something humiliating, perhaps; something you've failed at; something that, frankly, you'd just rather not discuss.

There's just so much baggage trailing behind "exercise." It's that thing that everyone is always going on about, as if it were the one thing that's standing between you and being . . . all kinds of things: "average size," "normal," "beautiful," "attractive" (as if any of those things had single definitions anyway or could infallibly produce such results for everyone!).

"Exercise" can, in fact, sound like just about the nastiest four-letter word around.

That's okay. There's no reason you have to use the word.

You can move your body without calling it anything at all. There's no reason in the world you have to name it. All you have to do is go out for that walk or head to the pool and have a swim or ride your bike or whatever. It's not "exercise." It's just moving around in the world, like people do.

If you do want to call the activity by a name, there are lots of names to choose from. For a number of years, the only word I could tolerate for my exercise was "bounce." As in "I'm going out for a bounce" or "I'm all stiff and I've been sitting in front of this computer too long—I need a bounce." For me, "bounce" worked not only because it was what I wanted to feel like I was doing—something playful and fun—but because for me, it held no baggage. Bouncing, as some of you may know, is what Tigger, of *Winnie the Pooh* fame, does, with his top made out of rubber and his bottom made out of springs. Who wouldn't want to bounce like Tigger?

You can, therefore, bounce if you'd like. Some people prefer to have a stomp or a surge or go on a walkabout. I have been known to be fond of "having a schvitz," the reference in this case not being to a steam bath—which is one of the meanings of the Yiddish word *schvitz*—but to sweating, the other meaning of *schvitz*. As a historian, I have a soft spot for "engaging in a spot of physical culture," "attending the gymkhana," and "taking my daily constitutional." Some of my friends have been known to chart their mileage against the peregrinations of the characters in *The Lord of the Rings,* whereupon each workout gets you further along the road to Mordor or back toward the Shire. Another friend "swam the English Channel," one half-hour stint in the pool at a time.

Call it "movement" if you want to. "Movement" is fine. Or just call it by the name of the activity you'll be engaging in: yoga or kayaking or pumping iron or playing hopscotch or walking on the beach. The point is, it doesn't matter what you call it. Call it "visiting Aunt Gertrude" if that makes you happy; you're not hurting anyone.

What matters is that you find language that lets you move without stumbling over what to call it. Whatever words help make moving your body feel comfortable or at least neutral to you are absolutely fine.

And now, if you'll excuse me, I think it's time for a bounce.

Health At Every Size

Another bit of highly useful language is the phrase "Health At Every Size." This is a phrase that's become a touchstone for size acceptance and especially for size-accepting fitness and health. It's the title of a fantastic book by nutritionist and researcher Linda Bacon (see the Resource Guide, page 197), in which she makes the rigorously researched, well-defended medical argument that your weight has much less to do with your overall health than is commonly assumed. Fat is not a deadly disease, and if all other factors are more or less equal—nutrition, stress, medical care, physical fitness, on so on—fat people and thinner people tend not to be too different in terms of their health outcomes. This argument has always been borne out beautifully by the lives of hundreds of thousands of fat people, but until Bacon's book came along, it has often been difficult to explain this convincingly to other people.

As Bacon demonstrates so well, it is, in fact, quite possible for people to be both fat and healthy. More to the point, there is no reason that people should not do what is in their power to improve and sustain their health regardless of their body size. Bacon's book, like this one, encourages you to take yourself and your needs seriously and to prioritize your health over your appearance, your clothes size, or any number on a scale.

Using "Health At Every Size," or "HAES," as a catchphrase can be useful to remind yourself of your body-practice priorities. It's also useful when you talk to fitness professionals, doctors, and others who either may have heard of the HAES approach or might be open to learning about this model. The fact that the HAES approach to health and well-being comes from within the biomedical community, is widely recognized as valid by medical authorities, and has the weight of a nice thick footnote-filled book behind it can go a long way toward convincing the resistant to work with you and not against you as you change your body practice and look for physical support and feedback that enhances your ability to reach your personal physical goals.

Getting the Right Feedback

After you've had some time to think about what you want to do with your-self and your body practice, it's time to start thinking about how you want to get feedback on your progress. There are a lot of great ways to do this and only two really bad ones, so let's get the bad ones out of the way first.

Bad Feedback Method: The Number on the Scale

The number on the scale doesn't measure anything that is particularly help-ful to you in terms of your body practice. It measures mass, and that is all. It does not measure virtue or goodness. It does not even measure health. It cannot tell you how muscular you are or whether you are more muscular now than you were three months ago. Muscle may weigh more than fat does, by volume, but your bathroom scale weighs all of you at the same time. Nor can the number on the scale tell you if your lungs are work-ing more effectively or your metabolism is self-regulating more efficiently.

The scale is not capable of imparting so much as a faint scintilla of a hint of information about your stamina, your flexibility, your skill, your reaction time, or how much you've improved your tennis game. The scale is a very limited device capable of one trick and one trick only, and, from the perspective of whether or not you're improving the functional capabilities of your body, it's not even a relevant trick.

Bad Feedback Method: The Skinny Jeans

That old pair of skinny jeans you haven't been able to fit into for God knows how long are just as limited and irrelevant a measure of your physical activity achievements as the number on the scale, and for identical reasons. Same goes for all their relatives, including the tape measure and the size of the clothes you wore in high school. Yes, yes, I know: every weight-loss product ad in the history of history depicts people fitting into smaller clothing sizes or shows a measuring tape wrapped snugly around something as evidence of "progress." But—and this is important—we are not talking about weight loss when we talk about movement; we're talking about increasing your physical capacity and ability, your confidence and pleasure in moving your body. These things are not the same as shrinking your body size and should not be confused.

Good feedback methods, on the other hand, exist in two basic types, objective and subjective. Objective forms of feedback that are worth your while include aerobic capacity, heart rate, and keeping notes on the quantitative aspects of the exercise you do, for instance, in terms of pounds/kilograms lifted for a particular exercise, or miles/kilometers per hour and the length of time that you walk or bike. Subjective feedback is the practice of asking yourself questions, making observations about what you perceive, and paying attention to how you feel when you are exercising.

Good Feedback Method: Aerobic Capacity

Aerobic capacity, sometimes known as VO_2max, is something that you can't easily measure yourself—a doctor would have to do this since it requires specialized equipment to measure the actual amounts of oxygen you take in and circulate through your blood while you're exercising. A personal trainer or a sports medicine professional can estimate it for you using a mathematical formula that derives a probable VO$_2$max figure from a series of heart-rate measurements made while you exercise.

Good Feedback Method: Heart Rate

Measuring your heart rate is easy. You'll need a clock or watch that can measure seconds. Place two fingers under the corner of your jaw until you feel the pulse in your carotid artery beneath your fingers. Count the number of beats that take place in six seconds. Multiply this number by ten, and you have the number of beats per minute (BPM) that is your current heart rate.

By testing your heart rate while you are doing various activities, you can find out roughly how hard your heart is working. Your BPM during exercise can be compared to the "target range" in which, statistically speaking, people in your age group are likely to receive the greatest benefit to cardiovascular functioning.

The American Heart Association gives the following target heart-rate ranges (as well as sample maximum healthy heart rates) as a general guideline. Note that these ranges change according to age range. Also be aware that there are some common drugs, such as beta blockers, that will prevent your heart rate from going as high as it would if you were unmedicated.

Age	Target Range	Maximum Healthy Heart Rate
20 years	100–170 BPM	200 BPM
25 years	98–166 BPM	195 BPM
30 years	95–162 BPM	190 BPM
35 years	93–157 BPM	185 BPM
40 years	90–153 BPM	180 BPM
45 years	88–149 BPM	175 BPM
50 years	85–145 BPM	170 BPM
55 years	83–140 BPM	165 BPM
60 years	80–136 BPM	160 BPM
65 years	78–132 BPM	155 BPM
70 years	75–128 BPM	150 BPM

Don't be surprised if, over time, your BPM for a particular activity at a particular intensity—let's say walking at 4 MPH—goes down. This is good, and it's exactly what you're trying to do! As your heart and lungs get better at what they do, and do it more efficiently, they will have to work less hard. Both at rest and while you're moving your body, your pulse rate will tend to stay lower and you won't start breathing heavily quite so easily. When this happens, you need only up the ante and work a little harder, let's say by bumping up your walking speed to 4.2 MPH or adding some hills and inclines to your walk, so that you can continue to keep the demand on your heart and lungs in the zone where it will encourage even greater efficiency.

Oh, and just in case you've just measured your heart rate while you're sitting here reading this, what you've just measured is called your *resting heart rate*, the number of times a minute your heart beats when you're not doing anything physical. A normal range for resting heart rate is between approximately sixty beats per minute and one hundred. Unusually low heart rate (bradycardia) and unusually high heart rate (tachycardia) can be signs of serious medical problems, so if your resting heart rate falls outside of this range, talk to your doctor.

Good Feedback Method: Quantitative Records

This is nothing more than keeping track of what you've done in quantitative terms—how many kilos or pounds of weight you lift for particular exercises, how far you walk at what speed, how many repetitions you do of an exercise or movement in a given session, how many laps of a pool of such-and-such length you swim in a given time period, and the like—and periodically looking back at your notes to see how things are progressing. This doesn't work for all forms of exercise, obviously. You can't so easily quantify exertion when you're doing aikido, say, or salsa dancing, but you can always keep track of how long you were moving your body, what kinds of things you learned in that aikido class, or how many songs in a row you danced to before you took a break, if you like.

One of the measurements physical trainers often use is to see how long it takes you to walk a mile (or a kilometer, if you prefer) going as fast as you can. Gauging how rapidly you can walk a given distance—if you want to get fancy you can call it the Rockport Walking Test, which is the name it has in exercise science—and testing again every so often to see how this changes is a nice tidy benchmark that is easy to measure.

Good Feedback Method: Subjective Experience

There are a number of questions that professional coaches and personal trainers use to help gauge how their clients are doing and what they are feeling during and after physical activity. Some have to do with how you perceive your exertion level, some have to do with how your body feels, and some have to do with your psychological state. You can use any or all of these as a way to check in with yourself in the moment as you move your body. You can do it informally without writing anything down or taking notes. Or you can use them as a self-interview in a more formal way, periodically asking yourself the questions and writing them down as a form of narrative record keeping. This can give you a really interesting picture of how you progress physically and mentally over time.

During Activity

- On a scale of 1 to 10, where 1 is "hardly making an effort" and 10 is "as hard as I possibly can," how hard am I working when I exercise?

- Are you breathing hard? A little, a lot, or not at all? More than is typical for you? Or less?

- Are you sweating? A little, a lot, or not at all? More than usual? Or less?

- How does this activity feel? Are there particular parts of your body that you are noticing? What are you feeling?

- How would you characterize your emotional state? Are there any ideas or thoughts that are coming up for you that seem noteworthy?

After Activity

- On a scale of 1 to 10, where 1 is "hardly making an effort" and 10 is "as hard as I possibly can," how hard would you say you worked, on average, today?

- Did any physical sensations come up that got your attention today? What were they? Were they fleeting or did they last a while?

- Did any emotional or psychological states come up that got your attention today? What were they? Were they fleeting or did they last a while?

- The following is a list of sensations or feelings that may arise in relation to physical exertion. Go down the list and see whether you feel more, less, or about the same in terms of each of these sensations or feelings as you did before you started: calm, agitated, energetic, fatigued, relaxed, enthusiastic, tired, happy, sad, angry, peaceful, worn out, depressed, upbeat, empowered.

Record keeping for feedback purposes can be done in many different ways. You can keep a notebook, chart things in a spreadsheet or chart, enter your data into an online exercise tracker, or record it in other ways. Some gyms, for instance, have computerized tracking available for their various exercise machines, where you need only enter an ID number before you begin exercising and everything you do will automatically be added to your personal chart. Other people like to use tools like pedometers, which count the number of steps you take while wearing them, or digital activity-tracking devices like the FitBit, which are basically fancy pedometers that are worn throughout the day or just during exercise and that have sensors that detect the amount and kind of activity you have accomplished while wearing them. You can just keep a body-practice journal. You can draw smiley faces on your calendar for every day you work physical activity into the day. The options are as varied, and as simple or detailed, as you want to make them.

You will need to experiment to find what level of record keeping works best for you. Some people like to keep track of everything they do every day. For others, this would be intolerable and would take all the enjoyment out of physical activity or worse, trigger obsessive-compulsive behavior. For some people, writing down benchmark figures once a week or every other week is enough to give them a sense of where they are, where they've been, and how things are going.

For some people, the convenience of online fitness and nutrition trackers (or software) is alluring. Many of these products have a very heavy-handed focus on weight loss and related information, such as calories expended. While some of us can put on our peril-sensitive sunglasses and ignore that sort of thing with relative ease, not everyone can do this comfortably. The implication that *of course* a fitness-tracking product user is—and should be!—interested in and prioritizing weight loss can be triggering, infuriating, or downright harmful to some people. If you try a fitness tracker and it makes you feel uncomfortable or bad or makes you feel forced to prioritize things you don't like, *don't use it*. Pencil and paper still work just fine, as does making your own computer spreadsheet or chart with customized fields that contain only the data you personally want to record.

Some people find that doing any record keeping at all where physical activity is concerned leaves a bad taste in the mouth, making them feel as though they are being judged or graded on their performance when they just want to be able to enjoy moving their bodies without pressure. If that describes you, don't panic. You don't have to keep written records, or any records at all, in order to be able to notice over time that movement is becoming easier, that you are feeling stronger, that you're more comfortable in your body, and all that good stuff. Sometimes, just noticing at random that you're doing something with ease that you couldn't do a few months ago is all the feedback you need.

INCENDIARY ACT #2

PAY REAL ATTENTION TO YOURSELF

When was the last time you paid real attention to yourself? I mean that you really focused on your physical and mental self long enough to take stock of where you are and how you're doing, physically and mentally, asking yourself what feels good or not so good, what's functioning badly or adequately or wonderfully, what you need help with, or what you're already good at?

Most of us don't do this very often. There's a lot of other stuff competing for our awareness, for one thing. Jobs and relationships and traffic and remembering to send that birthday card and oh crap, I forgot to get milk. . . . We've got a lot to juggle.

More insidiously, many of us also internalize the idea that paying attention to ourselves is bad. We might think it's selfish or that unless there's some immediate problem getting in our way, paying attention to

continued

ourselves is a waste of time. For women especially, there's also often the idea that only "good bodies" deserve attention and that bodies that aren't "good"—bodies that are lumpy or fat or pimply or plain or whatever—simply don't bear thinking about.

This is unhelpful, unfair, and unkind. It undermines us. It actively hurts us. If we're only willing to pay attention to ourselves when there's a crisis, then the only time we *get* that attention is when there's a crisis. This seems . . . counterproductive, to say the least.

For better or worse, we have bodies. We're obliged to live in them and with them every minute of every day. We spend more time in our bodies by far than we do in our cars, but are often less likely to pay attention to them: if a warning light is blinking on the dashboard or there's a weird noise when you accelerate the car, you pay attention. So why on earth wouldn't you pay attention to a warning sign like a sore elbow or a weird reaction when you drink soda with artificial coloring? You make a point of being aware of the kinds of things you might need to notice or do to keep your car running right . . . so how about for yourself?

Paying real attention to yourself, and taking the time to consciously go through your own body and mind to see what's going on in there, gives you the chance to troubleshoot, to plan, and to appreciate what's going well. You might come up with important things that will improve the way you function and feel. You might notice that "Oh hey, my lower back's all stiff. I should make a point of doing that Swiss ball exercise that stretches it out" or "I've been scared I'm going to fall ever since I tripped on that curb the other day. I need to find some way to improve my stability so I can relax about it."

Or you might, during your stock taking, realize that something you've been working on is paying off: "My moods really do seem more stable since I started walking at lunch; I guess the sunshine helps." Or you might just realize that you secretly feel pretty awesome and have found a great balance for your body and your brain . . . which is always a good thing to take note of, because it's harder to reproduce it if you don't know what you did in the first place.

In a world that teaches women to hate their bodies and tells them that their bodies aren't worthy unless they meet some arbitrary, narrow standard of "goodness" or "perfection," paying attention to your body as something that is totally worth your time and your care—and it is!—is radical, rebellious, and deeply cool.

What's So Bad About Boredom?

If you go by virtually everything you see in the fitness magazines and books and the things you hear from fitness professionals, you'd think that boredom was right up there with poverty, war, cancer, and interminable customer "service" telephone menus. Boredom, we're told, will kill your exercise practice dead. Boredom will yank the tender budding flower of physical well-being from your apathetic hands, leaving you dull and disappointed on the couch with Dr. Oz and some stale Doritos.

This is, not to put too fine a point on it, pretty much bullshit. Boredom isn't so bad as all that. We've all been bored before. We will all be bored again. We get bored at our jobs, driving our cars, reading the newspaper, watching TV. Tedium is tedious, but let's face it: there isn't a single one of us who hasn't figured out how to just knuckle down and get through doing something tedious when that's what's in front of us to do. Coping with boredom is part of being a grown-up. And although you may well decide it makes a reasonable excuse, boredom, all by itself, is not actually capable of forcing you to do anything you don't want to do.

I assume for the sake of argument that if you're reading this book, you are interested in having a successful and fruitful body practice. You're interested in getting stronger and fitter and more flexible, and you want to add things to your life like stamina and resilience and the freedom to play freely in the world you live in.

If that's the case, then boredom cannot possibly worry you too much. You have bigger fish to fry than whether or not you are bored for a little while every day or so while you get some exercise.

Personally, I have learned to welcome the sensation of boredom when I'm working out because boredom can actually provide opportunities that are relaxing and, dare I say it, even useful.

First of all, if you're feeling bored, you can just let your mind wander. Most of us don't get nearly as much time as we'd like to just think about things, ponder our way through thorny stuff that's going on in our lives, indulge in steamy daydreams, or imagine how good the living room will look with the right coat of paint and some new throw pillows. A nice boring repetitive form of exercise where you don't have to think too much about form or counting repetitions or making sure you don't run into a tree (I am very fond of the elliptical trainer for just these reasons) means you can just set yourself up, get going, and let your brain off its leash for a while.

You can also meditate while moving. There are whole branches of Buddhist meditation that are devoted to this, and of course many practitioners of yoga and martial arts (especially those like tai chi and qigong) also have meditative, spiritual aspects to their movement practices. Again, this is a place where having the activity be otherwise so familiar as to be rote and boring really helps: if you're going to meditate while you do it, your body has to be able to manage your movements without you needing to spend too much thought on it.

Feeling bored with your movement and your exercise routine is also a great time to check in on what you're doing and how you're doing in your body when you're moving around. Take the time to focus on some of the aspects you may not pay much attention to normally. How is your form? Is your body well aligned and moving easily and is your weight distributed well? Are you favoring one side of your body over the other or perhaps noticing some unevenness in your motions?

Be sure also to check on your intensity level. Do things feel too easy? Too hard? If you're either constantly fighting to get through your workout or constantly feeling as if you're not really being challenged, it can get old fast.

You can also take the opportunity afforded by boredom to ask yourself *why* you're bored. Are you not feeling challenged? Is the activity too repetitive? Do you want something more social, like a class, where you're exercising with other people? Have you just had enough of a particular activity and are chafing against doing yet more of it when you'd rather be doing something—anything—else? Is the scenery getting dull, and you're hankering for a change of venue? There are lots of different things that can be going on when we feel bored, after all, and lots of different ways you can make things less boring.

Or, y'know, you can just enjoy the sensation of knowing that in the midst of a challenging and often overstimulating life, you can go to the gym and do something that is simultaneously good for your body and good for your brain and that is, in its predictable ho-hum sameness, actually kind of reassuringly devoid of anything too exciting. Sometimes, a little bit of benevolent boredom is just what a right-thinking girl needs.

Give Yourself a Break

Sometimes, girl, you just have to give yourself a break. There are simply times when you're too stressed, too tightly scheduled, too sick, or just too fed up and in need of a good old-fashioned mental health day, and you need to put your body practice to one side.

How do you know when you really need a break? It's not actually all that hard to figure out. Ask yourself whether you really truly deep-down honestly feel like fifteen minutes is just too much.

Then pay attention to what comes up for an answer. If your answer is "Of course I could do fifteen minutes, and I probably should, but I don't feel like it," well, chances are that you're right and you probably should. If it's "Well, I could do fifteen minutes but I'm afraid that the same guy who was such a loud, aggressive douche on Tuesday is going to be at the gym again and I just don't want to have to deal with it," then the issue isn't that you need a break from your body practice so much as that you need a break from dealing with Douchey Dude. It might be worth reassessing to see whether you have the wherewithal to just go, give Douchey Dude the finger (in your head or otherwise), and get your fill-up of tasty, tasty movement endorphins. After all, he's a douche! Are you really going to let him run the show? Of course not.

On the other hand, if you ask yourself this question and the answer is "Oh God—I couldn't even be vertical for fifteen whole minutes," then chances are good you're sick enough that you really need to just go lay down and not worry about the gym. If it's "I haven't had fifteen minutes to myself in so long I forget what it's like," then I strongly suspect you're chronically overbooked and you need to go somewhere quiet and stare at a wall for a while. And if your answer is "I'm freaking out at the drop of a hat today, and I really need to not have anything bad happen or I may completely drop my beads," well, we all have those days and if once in a while you decide that it is really just too much to deal with, that's okay.

There's nothing wrong with taking a few days or even a few weeks—or months, if you have to—off from an active body practice now and then. Sometimes it's medically necessary. Other times life intervenes. And while there are some kinds of life stress where it really helps to be able to take an hour off every so often and go for that walk or swim or whatever it is, and while it is also true that many people find that regular physical movement helps keep their mood more stable, there are also times when that's not true and maybe not even possible.

It doesn't hurt anybody if you occasionally take a break from active pursuit of your body practice. You may find that you lose enough of the tangible physical benefits of it, such as more stable mood or energy or blood sugar levels, that you want to keep your breaks as short as possible, and if so, that's okay. There are reasons that many people sidelined by injury or illness actually go out of their way to find less-strenuous and safe ways to get back to movement sooner rather than later. On the whole, the worst thing that a break can do is to make you lose a little ground or make you feel rusty when you go back to your body practice, and those are things that are easily made up for once you're back in the swing of things.

Take a break if you're injured. Take a break if you're sick. Take a break if you're so stressed out that getting some exercise doesn't feel like it helps but only makes things tighter and more wound up and frantic. Take a break if you're feeling too fragile or if you're hitting an uncommonly rough patch with your mental health and exercising seems to make it worse rather than better.

Don't worry that you'll take a break and never start up again. Having that worry is, in actual fact, a pretty good guarantee that it won't happen. (It's when you start going "Oh, what's one more day? I'll start up again tomorrow. . . " that you start to run into trouble.) Tell yourself that just for today—or just for the week, or for however long it takes you to be able to breathe through your nose again, or for however long it is that the doctor tells you to stay off that sprained ankle—it's okay to not worry about it. If you're going to take a break, it might as well be a real one, without guilt or angst. Knowing when to take a break, and being able to let yourself off the hook when you need it, is part of your body practice too.

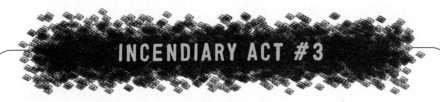

INCENDIARY ACT #3

HAVE YOUR OWN REASONS TO DO THE THINGS YOU DO

Just because you live in a culture that yowls so incessantly about movement and weight loss that you'd think "dietandexercise" was a single word, it doesn't mean you have to sing from that same dull old hymnal.

You are 100 percent entitled to have your very own reasons to do the things you do in this life, and that very much includes the reasons you decide to move your body and the ways you decide to move it.

Just because other people may assume that you're walking, swimming, unicycling, skateboarding, kayaking, playing wheelchair basketball, snowshoeing, or kickboxing because you want to lose weight or "look better" (or whatever euphemism du jour is on the menu) doesn't mean you are—or that you have to want to.

Ditto for other serious-sounding agendas. Sure, exercising is good for you and all. It's great for your blood pressure and your heart rate and blood oxygenation and muscle condition and bone mineral density and insulin sensitivity and so on. Maybe you're interested in that stuff and maybe you aren't. Maybe those kinds of things are some of the goals you have for your exercising and maybe they're not. Or maybe they're just not the ones you want to have to think about all the damn time.

It's fine if you have Serious-Business Grown-Up reasons to exercise. But it's also fine if you don't or if those are things you only think about sometimes.

It's completely okay if you get your hula hoop on just because it's fun, you know. It's utterly fine if you go hiking because you geek out about trees and rocks, or if you play softball because you like to hang out with your friends on the team. It's 100 percent acceptable to be jazzed about going to the gym because the elliptical trainer is where you meditate. It's totally reasonable to love dojo time primarily because of the satisfying *thud* when you knock someone to the mat. If you like running your errands by bicycle because it's so much easier to find a place to park, that's all the reason you need. And it is always thoroughly cool to enjoy moving your body just because it feels good.

Your body. Your movement. Your reasons. Your life. That's all you need.

Getting Back on the Horse

So you've taken a break from moving your body regularly, getting exercise, doing that whole thing. Whether intentionally, unintentionally, because of an injury, because you just had a world-beating case of the fuckits for a while, it doesn't matter. What matters is that you're ready, now, to get back to it.

So let's get one thing out of the way: if you're feeling guilty or regretting that you took a break because now it's just so hard to go back to it, just let that go. You took a hiatus because you took a hiatus, you did what you did, and that's all water under the bridge—no matter why you did it, no matter how long you did it for, no matter what. Neither guilt nor regret are going to get your blood pumping and your muscles warm and happy, so to hell with them and welcome back!

Now that you're back on your feet, the next step is to try to figure out just how those feet are doing. Unless your break was quite short—a week or two at most—you can't assume that you're going to be able to just leap right back into activity at the same level that you were at before your break. Start slowly, warm up thoroughly, and only then push yourself a little to find out where you stand, what your capacity for movement looks and feels like at the moment. Follow the techniques in the 80 Percent Rule section (page 138), pushing yourself to the point of what yoga teacher Abby Lentz calls "sweet discomfort," then backing away to something sustainable from which you can build.

All other things being equal, any lost ground can be regained. If you are recovering from an injury or illness, this may take a little longer than it would otherwise, but improvements can still be made. Generally speaking, ground lost to a hiatus from active body practice is not lost, just temporarily misplaced. You'll get it back, and more.

At this point, you may need to return to the no-regrets and no-guilt part. Losing ground can be an emotional blow, but there's nothing to be done for it but to start again where you are right now. Don't try to add a lot of new or extra activity when you're just resuming your active body practice. The impulse to make up for lost time is understandable, but push too hard too fast and it's going to be counterproductive. Your body hasn't been asked to do as much lately, and it has adjusted to that state of affairs. Insisting that your body suddenly go from zero to sixty just because you've decided to stomp your foot down on the gas right this instant is a great way to hurt yourself or burn yourself out in a hurry. A good general rule is to give yourself the same amount of time to get back to where you were when you left off as you took time away from being active. Take your time, get back to where you were, and *then* worry about adding to or making big changes in your routines. And if you're worried that other people might notice that you're not quite up to the level that you used to be, and may be unkind or mocking about it, read on.

CHAPTER 2

Chub, Sweat, and Jeers

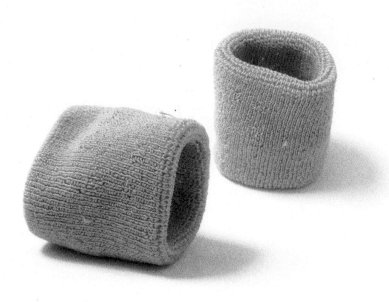

"Hell is other people," said the French philosopher Jean-Paul Sartre, and he wasn't even a fat guy. Dealing with criticism, commentary, judgment, and sometimes outright mockery and humiliation about your size while you're trying to do right by your body is really tough to take. That's why it's good to know that you're not alone or without resources, and that you don't have to let other people's bad manners get in the way of your having a body practice that feels good in every possible way.

That Target on Your Back

It's unfair, it's exasperating, it's outrageous, it's undeserved, and it's nevertheless true: when you move in the world as a fat woman, people feel entitled to comment. They'll comment on what you look like. They'll comment on what you do and on what you don't do. Most of all, they'll comment on what they *believe* is true about you, whether or not it has any bearing on reality.

Sometimes these comments are easy enough to ignore. Sometimes they're impossible to ignore. Some of it is laughable, and some of it is unbelievably nasty and painful. As fat women, we often seem like we have targets on our backs. It's wrong, it's undeserved, and it's miserable.

This is particularly pertinent to the unapologetic fat girl because one of the things many fat women do in an attempt to avoid harassment and abuse is to avoid physical activity and exercise. As a result, many of us avoid getting physical where anyone else might see, particularly in places like gyms and swimming pools, yoga studios and public parks, where our bodies are likely to be exposed to view.

It can be especially difficult, as a fat woman, to enter into spaces where we know (or strongly suspect) that a particular athletic and/or slim body aesthetic that our bodies don't fit is the standard to which people's bodies will be held. It can be hard to even consider wearing a swimsuit or bike shorts or tank tops, no matter how appropriate or comfortable those would be. We may fear that the further away we are from the ideal or the expected body, and the more of it people can see, the more painful criticism there will be.

We may be afraid that if we lack competence or ability, this too will leave us open to unfriendly fire. No one wants to be seen as a caricature of a puffing, panting, sweaty, red-faced fattie. No one wants to have their lack of prowess in some activity become something that other people focus on or, worse yet, ridicule. No one wants to be seen fumbling, flailing, or looking like a rank beginner. We all fear it. Some of us have excellent reasons to fear it, too, having learned early on that we would be bullied and tormented in athletic contexts.

No wonder so many fat people—women and men alike—are so hesitant to get physically active. What kind of masochist do you have to be to put yourself out there to be nonconsensually tormented at random by strangers? For many of us, after all, this has been a thing we've experienced, and we aren't keen on doing it again.

No one deserves to learn, or God forbid be actively taught, that she is an unworthy and unacceptable human being who should not participate in a full and physical life. No one should be so bullied and harassed for what they are that they learn to voluntarily shrink their lives and limit their activities, refuse to let themselves do things they want and need to do, or refrain from doing things that bring them pleasure and health in order to cut down on the amount of cruelty they encounter.

And no one should have to learn the bitter lesson that even if you do these things to minimize yourself, it doesn't actually protect you. Circumscribing your life to avoid harassment doesn't actually make the harassment vanish; it just means that you're circumscribing your life *and* being harassed. No one, no matter what they look like, actually deserves to be the target of opportunistic nastiness, not even if inwardly, they fear they really do deserve it. They don't. *You* don't.

Knowing that, and believing it, is the first step in dealing with it. You're not wrong to want to move your body. You're not wrong to have a body that doesn't conform to what other people might prefer to see. (Who died and put them in charge anyway?) You are a human being in a human body, and your body has its needs just like every other. Physical activity is one of those needs. If you wouldn't apologize for having a drink of water, you shouldn't even be thinking about apologizing for moving your body. There is no wrong way to have a body! The wrongness lies with the people who refuse to simply live and let live.

The second step in dealing with the fear of bullying and harassment is, for better or worse, to just get out there and get in the game anyway. Hiding your fatness and not going out and doing what you want to do has never magically made other people's bad behavior vanish. All it does is prevent you from going out and doing what you want to do. Our big weapon, as people who want better lives for ourselves and others, is doing exactly what the haters don't want us to do: showing up and doing things.

The more you behave like you have the right to exist in the world without interference, the less others will question it. The power of a fait accompli is astonishing. The more people see fat bodies moving and being physical and doing whatever makes them happy in the world, without apology and without shame, the more they get used to seeing that and thinking of it as normal.

Will you occasionally encounter harassment? Probably. Will you occasionally encounter fat-phobic assholery? Probably. But that isn't anything you haven't dealt with before, you know. What's more, there are ways to deal with it so that it doesn't break your stride. Here are some things that help:

- **Be bored.** Anti-fat harassment is, frankly, boring. No one ever comes up with anything new. It's always the same tedious, predictable, tired, lazy crap, and I am willing to bet you've seen and heard it all before. Feel free to just roll your eyes and keep on doing what you were doing before someone decided to take some time out of their busy day to be tediously, predictably, and lazily obnoxious at you. If they get cranky at not getting a reaction and get in your face about it, just tell them that you're aware you're fat, thanks, and that you have things to do and it's time for them to get out of your way.

- **Be willing to tell them what they're doing.** It's amazing how effective it can be to simply say "That was rude" and walk away. Informing people that they are behaving badly, without behaving badly yourself, lets you name the wrongdoing, call the person out so they aren't just getting away with it, and still keep the moral high ground. Steer clear of calling people names, if you possibly can. This is about behaviors, not personalities. Heaven knows they don't have any personal investment in *you*; they're just indulging themselves in crappy behavior at a convenient target, so call it like you see it. Should you be met with a "but you're *fat*"—as if it legitimized their nastiness—you can always say "Yes I am, and that was rude."

- **Stare.** A level, unflinching, completely flat stare can unnerve even cocky teenaged boys. Channel your inner Head Librarian and just stare at the person until you melt holes through their head or they leave the room, whichever comes first. You can stare while you continue your workout, by the way. It needn't slow you down.

- **Shame them.** As with calling out bad behavior, this is best done very simply and succinctly. If someone is nasty or abusive, you can simply look them in the eye and say "Shame on you. That was unnecessary and unkind, and you know better." Because people *do* know better. They know better than to judge, they know better than to give unsolicited commentary, and they know better than to say unkind things. After all, *you* know better than that. And so do they. There's no reason they shouldn't feel ashamed of making the choice to let their uncivil impulses run the show.

- **Ignore it.** Harassment is boring, tedious, uses resources that you have better uses for, and does not improve your life in any way . . . so why pay attention? Yes, sometimes people intentionally make it as disruptive as they possibly can so that they know they've gotten your attention, but a lot of the time they don't. And if they don't, why bother giving them the satisfaction of having you pay attention to them? If you wouldn't shrink from brushing off a mosquito, you shouldn't have a single reservation about blowing off someone who, like a mosquito, only wants to irritate and annoy you and feed off your discomfort.

INCENDIARY ACT #4

DON'T MAKE YOURSELF RESPONSIBLE FOR OTHER PEOPLE'S BAD BEHAVIOR

You know the hoary old formula we trot out when something bad happens, the one that runs "Well, if you just weren't so such-and-so . . . " then "it" wouldn't have happened—as in "If you weren't so blonde, people wouldn't think you were stupid" or "If you weren't quite so large, people wouldn't stare or make comments"?

Of course you do; we all know that formula. It's where we undermine our friends and ourselves by working backward from a moment of abusive behavior to see if we can figure out why it happened. We superstitiously think, if only we don't do whatever it is, it'll make us safe. The only problems here are that it won't—because abusive behavior is abusive. Abuse is never justified, even when people try to make excuses for it.

Another name for this is *blaming the victim*, as in "If you weren't wearing such a short skirt, he wouldn't have tried to rape you." It's a lazy, insidious mental habit. We indulge in it partly for legitimate reasons, when we are trying to understand why someone would be abusive. But we also do it because it's much easier to blame the victim, even when that means blaming yourself, than it is to confront abuse and hold accountable people who are behaving badly.

A lot of us internalize this dynamic so much that we do it to ourselves reflexively. "If only I were two sizes smaller," we think, "then those women at yoga wouldn't laugh behind my back." Easier to blame yourself and go home feeling crappy than to call them on it and tell them off and take the risk that they might be mean to you all over again, or worse yet, laugh at you.

But just because it's easier doesn't mean it's right.

The only person who is responsible for being a jackass is the person who is being the jackass. Anyone can make an *excuse* for being a jackass. But that doesn't mean they aren't still being a jackass.

Anyone can make excuses for being small-minded, petty, cruel, parochial, or abusive. But that doesn't mean they're not or that their behavior is justified.

You are not responsible for what other people allow to go on inside their heads. They are.

You are not responsible for what other people allow to come out of their mouths. They are.

You are not responsible for other people's actions. They are.

I don't care how fat you are. I don't care how funny-looking you are. I don't care how old or disabled or poor or underemployed or uneducated you are. I want you, right here, right now, to *stop holding yourself responsible for other people's bad behavior.* You are not obligated to tolerate or indulge cruelty or nastiness of any sort just because you are not perfect in every way. *No one is perfect.* And no one should be made to feel that their imperfections mean they must take responsibility for the fact that someone else is nasty, cruel, or abusive.

Voices in Your Head

What's more difficult than dealing with crappy and unsolicited commentary from other people? Why, that would be coping with your own internal Greek chorus of criticism, self-loathing, perfectionism, and unrealistic expectations, of course!

There's probably no one alive who doesn't experience some version of this. I've certainly never met anyone who didn't have a somewhat idealized internal version of themselves in their heads or who didn't experience at least a little bit of angst or anguish over the distance they perceived between the idealized version and the real live everyday model. It's not limited to us fat girls, but we do get an extra-hefty dose of shame, guilt, and other nasties connected with a lifetime's worth of other people's idealized notions of what our bodies "should be."

We construct our internal obstacle courses in lots of ways, out of lots of different materials. As you work on your body practice, try to be conscious of what the hurdles look like in your internal obstacle course. Pay attention to what themes come up. If you can recognize the kind of obstacle you're facing and be realistic about the nature of the obstacle in question, you stand a better chance of finding a way to negotiate a way around, over, or even through it.

For example, we may find that we have retained a tendency to judge our physical fitness by the sneering standards of a sadistic junior high school gym teacher. Can't run around that track without huffing and puffing? Still terrified of team sports? Can't do a chin-up? These things don't actually mean you're a fitness failure, no matter how loudly your internal gym teacher yells and blows that whistle. Why not brainstorm some ways that you can track your fitness progress that don't feel so yucky and punitive? There's no reason that you can't judge your own fitness on the basis of other things, like how you feel after you hike a mile in the woods or how many days in a row you've managed to go for a bike ride after work. Try "Getting the Right Feedback" (page 29) for some much better ways of gauging your fitness and your progress, ways that won't make you feel like the most miserable part of eighth grade all over again.

Or perhaps you're feeling like you must be doing it wrong unless you combine exactly the right mix of exercises in exactly the right order. If you aren't getting your heart rate to exactly the right percentage of your maximum for the right amount of time or doing the right number of sit-ups, it's all for naught.

It's easy to fall into the trap of thinking that unless you're following some established orthodoxy, you must be doing something wrong. Why not cut yourself a little slack and give your body credit for the millions of years of evolution that went into making it into something that thrives on a huge variety of types of physical movement? It helps to keep in mind that our ancestors, very probably including your grandparents, did not know any of this stuff that is supposedly true about how you're supposed to move your body for maximum whateverness. They just walked a lot and carried things around from place to place and did a lot of manual labor because that's what they had to do to survive, and, oddly enough, they got along without a single exercise specifically targeting their upper abdominals. Moving your body in some ways is better than moving your body in no ways. The goal of an active body practice is, ultimately, just giving your body what it needs to be happy, and that can look like an awful lot of things.

You may also be running hard into a lot of ideas and superstitions about what exercise is supposed to make your body look like. Many people do, and in fact, it's hard to avoid given all the messages that we get that regular exercise is the magic wand that can force your body to look exactly like you want it to. You may feel like it's not worth spending the time exercising if you aren't instantly transformed into a size 10, or like you're just not getting anywhere because you don't look any more like the girl from the track and field team who won the attention of the person you had a crush on when you were in college. The fact is that exercising is not going to make you into something totally different from what the directions encoded in your DNA will allow. It doesn't do that for *anybody*. It can't. You might as well expect it to do your taxes and pick out your mother's birthday present. Exercise is only going to make you into a more physically competent, strong, flexible, and resilient version of yourself. Your body may change (see page 152), but it's only ever going to be your body with its particular collection of attributes and capacities.

Maybe you're even having trouble convincing yourself to go to the gym because, shockingly enough, you *like* it, and it just doesn't jibe with your self-image to suddenly be a person who enjoys doing the kind of stuff that everyone's always been trying to tell you to do so you'll lose weight. Maybe you have a real problem with feeling like you must appear, to others, to be buying into the whole shtick about how fat people should exercise all the time. Maybe you're insecure about what it says about you that you're suddenly changing your ways in terms of your body practice. This is all real stuff and can be surprisingly tricky to negotiate. Having sturdy reasons of your very own for your body practice helps a lot. (See "Change Is Inevitable," page 152.) Revisiting why you're doing what you're doing with your body practice, what you're getting out of it, and why it matters to you to continue to do it helps you keep from feeling like you're having whiplash.

Whatever the internal obstacles you're running up against, there are ways to negotiate with them. We all have our issues with our bodies, with exercise, and with other people's reactions to our bodies and our physical activity. Look the obstacles in the eye and remember that you're the boss, not them. You're bigger than they are, and they don't get to tell you what to do. It's okay. Just keep moving. You're going to be fine.

Opinions Are Like Assholes

One of the best pieces of advice anyone ever gave me was this: Opinions are like assholes. Everyone's got one. Most people are quite fond of their own, especially in private. Yet they're not really something that should be waved around too much in public. When they are, it's okay to ignore them, because showing them off, unsolicited, is actually kind of rude.

Virtually every single thing that any other person tells you about your body, your weight, your size, or your appearance is in fact an opinion. With the exception of things that can be measured objectively—your blood pressure, for instance, your blood sugar level, and so on—everything else is an opinion, an interpretation, or a judgment.

This means that "Your weight is not proportionate to your height" is an opinion. Clearly your weight does exist in some proportion to your height. Mathematically speaking, it is inevitable that this is so. However, calling something "proportionate" implies that there is a *proper* proportion for this relationship and that all the rest of the possibilities are *improper*. And *that*, my friend, is an opinion, a value judgment, an interpretation—not a fact.

The fact, in this case, is that your weight and your height have a mathematical relationship to one another and that relationship may or may not have anything to do with whether or not you feel comfortable, happy, healthy, energetic, and good in your own body.

Similarly, what this means is that exercise instructors (whether they be books or videos or actual human beings live and in front of you) who tell you what you *should* be doing with your body, how intensely you should be doing it, or how many times are also providing you with opinions and recommendations, but not with ironclad, irrefutable facts. Here's a real fact for you: any exercise is better than no exercise, as far as the human body is concerned. But more exercise or more intense exercise is *not* always better than less. Sometimes our bodies need time to level up. Sometimes we have injuries or illnesses that mean we just shouldn't push too hard.

Someone else's opinion of what they think is going to be best for you, physically speaking, is not always what *is* going to be best for you. It is up to you to remember that recommendations about your fitness are just that, recommendations. They're not commandments carved in stone. You have to evaluate them and decide whether or not those opinions make sense to you, whether they work for you, and whether you think they're sound.

And this all goes double, triple, five thousand times for all the little voices that filter in from all around us, the ones that are always there to offer some sort of negative comment on how slow we're going, or how we look in those bike shorts, or what that person over there must be thinking about us, or whether we're working hard enough at the gym.

Take that step back. Think how inappropriate it would be if someone just walked up and mooned you, forced you to deal with the unsolicited, unrefusable sight of their bare butt. The sudden, unrefusable presence of an unsolicited opinion is not so different, really. It's perfectly all right if your reactions to opinions are exactly the same: You have every right to be offended. You don't have to pay attention. And they do not have to have a voice in shaping your reality.

When Compliments Aren't

Sometimes what sounds like a compliment on the surface doesn't feel very complimentary.

Sometimes this is because a lot of us have a really hard time taking a compliment. Especially if we don't feel good about ourselves, it's pretty hard to accept it if someone else expresses a positive opinion. We may behave as if there's an unwritten rule that if *we* don't approve of some aspect of ourselves, then no one else gets to either.

But sometimes we're not just being contrary. When we're being complimented for something that we honestly don't think is a good thing, it can be hard to take. For example, many people, of a wide range of body sizes, have had the experience of losing weight because they are sick or grieving, only to not know what to do or how to take it later on when someone compliments them on losing weight. They didn't intend to lose any weight, and the weight loss was a side effect of being utterly miserable. These "compliments" can feel like we're being told that it was a good thing that we were in such desperate straits.

If this sort of thing happens to you, it's okay to tell people "Hey, I understand that you mean well, but that wasn't the compliment you thought it was, and here's why." They won't magically know it. You have to tell them.

Sometimes compliments feel like someone's just nonchalantly leaned an elbow right on top of a big red button marked "DO NOT PRESS." I personally want to spit tacks and broken glass every time someone strikes up a conversation with me at the gym with the purpose of praising the fat girl for being at the gym and telling me how great it is that I'm there to "get in shape," as if they knew the first thing about me or why I'm in the gym, what my goals are, or what my exercise history is like—as if it were any of their business! *Round is a shape,* I want to snarl. *I've been coming to this gym five or six times a week for years, which you would know if you spent more time here yourself.*

I mostly do not say these things because I try to be polite. But I will often say something milder that will get some of the same point across, like "Oh, you must be new here; I've never run into you before. Have a great workout!" Defusing the compliment in a way that makes it gently but firmly clear that the compliment was not actually appropriate is an excellent and useful technique. Casualness is key. You aren't making a big deal out of something that isn't a big deal, and neither should they.

Of course, sometimes compliments just aren't really compliments. Underhanded compliments are, for better or worse, nothing new or unusual. "You sure do work out a lot; you must have lost a lot of weight," is one I've heard about from several fat athlete friends. The presumption, of course, being that of course exercise produces weight loss, so either the person has lost weight or the whole system's broken, and that would be intolerable. You know how it goes.

With these, the only really good answer is not to give the underhanded compliment giver any traction. "Huh, yeah, I guess I do work out a lot more than some folks," works better than trying to defend your weight, regardless of what it is or whether it's changed. The best responses to underhanded compliments are ones that leave the conversation with nowhere to go.

When I am trying to decide how to deal with a compliment, whether it seems sincere or underhanded, I try to remind myself of this: a compliment is just another way to register an opinion. And opinions are, as noted in the previous section, kind of like assholes. Some you're okay with, but most you really don't need to know about.

You do not *have* to take a compliment. You really don't. And there are times you shouldn't. That's as it should be. Other people don't get to be passive-aggressive at you just because you're fat.

Concern Trolling

You may or may not have heard the phrase "concern trolling," but it's a good bet you've experienced the phenomenon. Concern trolling is when someone appears to be concerned for your health or welfare, but only until they can catch you with your guard down so they can go after you about your weight, size, or whatever they presume is true about your fitness levels and general health.

This is the old "I'm just worried about your health" trick. When "I'm just worried about your health" is an insinuation that you *aren't* worried about it and implies that you must be negligent just because you're not thin, you have entered the realm of concern trolling. Sometimes "concern" is the foot someone jams in the door so you can't close it against condescension, presumption, invasiveness, and, at times, outright abuse. Like backhanded compliments, concern trolling is a passive-aggressive technique that can fly under your self-protective radar and let people get their hooks into you despite your best efforts to keep these kinds of interactions at bay.

Because of the expression of concern, concern trolling can be harder to disregard than other forms of negative comments. We legitimately fear and worry about bad outcomes like injuries, illness, and pain. And this is precisely why concern trolling works so well. Reasonably enough, we want to avoid bad experiences! Even when you are pretty secure in your own physical body and have a good sense of what you're about, concern trolling can make it all too easy to doubt yourself and think that maybe the person talking to you knows something you don't. And you know, they might . . . but most of the time, they don't.

Concern trolling is particularly relevant with regard to exercise. For various reasons, people can be threatened by a fat person's decision to become more active. They may feel like it makes them look bad by comparison for not exercising more or not being more fit themselves. They may have deeply rooted prejudices about fat people not deserving to exercise or it not being appropriate. Or they might just be uncomfortable with the idea that you're doing something they haven't seen fat people do very much. People sometimes react very poorly to having their worldview challenged, even if their worldview is actually shamefully narrow. This, however, is not your problem to solve.

People who feel threatened like this are sometimes wont to approach a fat exerciser with concern-trolling tactics like "Running at your size? Aren't you worried about knee injury?" or "You should be careful. I read in the paper that someone your size had a heart attack while at the gym the other week."

INCENDIARY ACT #5

DON'T DO THE ASSHOLES' JOB FOR THEM

Many of us live with a lot of fear about our bodies. We fear that our bodies will be found lacking and therefore we will not be found desirable, worthwhile, employable, lovable, respectable. . . . The list goes on and on. More often than many of us would like to admit, we let fear box us in, limit us, and circumscribe our lives.

This happens in many different ways. We may fear that if other people see our bodies, they'll mock us. As a result we might avoid going sleeveless, wearing shorts, wearing bright colors, putting on swimsuits, going to the beach. Sometimes we even avoid leaving the house.

We may also fear that if we struggle with physical things, people will ridicule us or take advantage of our weakness. So we just don't sign up for that Pilates class we've been interested in, convinced that everyone else there will be a combination ballet dancer-model-contortionist and they'll all huddle together at one side of the room in their immaculate, stylish exercise clothes whispering and staring at us. We don't set up a session with that personal trainer because the thought that she might be mean and make us cry like those trainers on *Biggest Loser* is more than enough to make us not want to find out what that experience is like. Maybe we don't even go for a walk with our friends because we don't want them to give us a hard time if we're not able to go as fast or as far as they want or to get frustrated with us if we need to sit down sometimes and take a break.

In short, we're afraid that someone's going to be an asshole to us because of something having to do with our bodies. So we try to minimize the possibility of assholery by exposing ourselves as little as we possibly can.

The problem with this is that every time we let this fear get the upper hand and we shut ourselves down or cut off our own possibilities, we're doing the assholes' job for them. What these jerks are really trying to do is to control other people, to silence them and humiliate them and get them to dance to whatever unpleasant tune they might happen to want to play. They want to feel powerful. The way they try to get power for themselves is by making other people feel powerless by taking away their options and their choices. When we limit our own options and choices and preemptively make ourselves powerless, we're just cutting out the middleman. We're doing the assholes' work for them.

There's no advantage in doing this. Offering yourself up as a sacrifice does not, unfortunately, buy you immunity. Assholes are going to rear their ugly heads in your life now and then no matter what you do. Oppressing, scaring, and browbeating yourself only means that you're oppressed, scared, and browbeaten, *plus* you sometimes have to deal with assholes.

People who are prone to being assholes do not need or deserve your help.

So why not take that Pilates class, go for that walk, and set up an interview with that personal trainer? Put on a swimsuit and make like a mermaid. Pop on a pair of bike shorts and a tank top and take that Schwinn for a spin. Or just walk out your own damn front door with your head high like the world belongs to you, too.

(It does, you know.)

Quit doing the assholes' job for them. They're going to be assholes anyway. You don't have to make it easier for them.

Whatever the comment may be, whatever flavor of trumped-up concern is being displayed, the proper answer is always to *trust yourself first*. You are the person who lives in your body. You are the person on the ground, as it were, and you will always be the very first person who will have an opportunity to notice whether there is legitimate reason for concern for your health or well-being. You are the person who knows whether things feel bad or good, whether you feel like something hurts in a bad way or whether you're just pushing yourself in ways that are making you stronger. That other person is not the boss of you!

With that in mind, you can practice simply saying, "I appreciate the concern; everything's just fine over here." Repeat that often enough, in the very same monotone, and even the most dogged of concern trolls will eventually give up and slink off . . . and if trolls carp about how dismissive you were, well, I suppose life's tough when someone refuses to let them behave like a jerk. Because you know what? Everything really *is* a whole lot more likely to be just fine when people aren't being jerks, amazingly enough.

Get Out of My Way

Sometimes you just have to tell other people to get out of your way.

You're entitled to get out in the world and move your body. It doesn't matter how much you weigh, what you look like, or what other people think. You, yes you, are completely within your rights to get out there and walk, jump, swim, climb, run, hang glide, scuba dive, and line dance as much as you like. In fact, you're entitled to as much movement as you damn well please. Cross my heart, hope to die—I promise. You really are.

Many people forget this. It's easy to understand why. Society loves to tell us all about the things that fat people, and especially fat women, shouldn't be doing or don't deserve to do. People can be cruel and crass and nasty and unpleasant, punitive and callous and rude, all in the name of trying to keep you in whatever it is that they think your place should be. The attempt to avoid the abuse and the criticism by simply avoiding doing the things that seem to trigger the abuse is totally logical, and forgetting that you have the right to play freely in the world is a logical extension of this avoidance.

It's also unnecessary. There is no rule anywhere that says that a human being only gets to do the kinds of things human beings do if they meet certain stringent weight requirements. And going out in the world and doing things, moving your body in all the various ways that you might want to move it, is a human thing.

That's why, for anyone who struggles with the notion that they genuinely deserve to be allowed to move their bodies freely and happily in the world, I strongly recommend using one very simple phrase: "Get out of my way."

You can say it to people who try to tell you what you're not supposed to be doing. Why should they get in the way of your doing what you want and need to do?

You can say it to the voices in your head that try to tell you it's not worth it, that you'll be laughed at, that you're just being a fool. Why should they get to tell you what to do? They're not the boss—you are.

You can definitely say it to anyone, anywhere, who tells you that you won't be able to do what you want to do. How would they know? And besides, even if what you've set out to do proves impossible, why shouldn't you have the fun of trying?

"Get out of my way" works because it states, very clearly, that you have something to do. You have a way you are headed. And someone else is interfering. It's not *you* who is the interloper here. It's not *you* who is disturbing things or being out of line. Someone's in your way. And they need to get out of it.

Haters gonna hate, as the kids say these days, and party poopers are gonna poop. Let them do it somewhere else. Get out of my way.

Teachable Moments

As fat people, we often end up feeling like we must additionally agree to be teachers if we want to be treated with respect. Because so many people's beliefs about fat people and our bodies and our experiences are built primarily out of stereotypes and presumptions, we often feel compelled to teach people the truth about our lives simply in order to be able to get them to treat us with basic respect.

- No, we have to explain, fat people don't all constantly eat fast food.
- Yes, there is a lot of diversity in the shapes and sizes of bodies; fat people don't all look alike.

- No, not every fat person is fat for the same reasons.
- Yes, fat people eat salads.
- No, not every fat person has health problems.
- Yes, fat people do have lovers and spouses and sex lives, thank you very much.
- No, it's not impossible to be a happy person and a fat one, too.
- Yes, fat people go to the gym.

Sometimes, it's worth taking advantage of the "teachable moment" and spending the time and the effort to try to build a bridge with someone. But as the old saying runs, "You can lead a horse to water, but you can't make it drink." Not all teachable moments end up teaching anyone anything useful. Some of the time all anyone gets taught is that you can't teach someone something they're not willing to learn. That's a drain on your resources and a waste of your time.

For all these reasons, it's a good idea to remember that when it comes to size issues generally and size and fitness specifically, it is not necessarily your responsibility to teach people. No matter how ignorant others may be, how presumptuous they may be about you or people like you, no matter how uncharitable their views or flat-out wrong their information, other people are ultimately not your responsibility. Unless someone's paying you to teach them differently, it's really okay to let ignorant people be ignorant unless you genuinely feel like taking on the task of teaching. (Not like you could teach them all anyway. There is probably as much ignorance out there as there is oxygen.)

When it comes to fat and exercise, the best way to teach is often by example. Instead of telling someone that you exercise, just let them see you do it. Rather than wasting your precious gym time defending your right to wear bike shorts, just wear them, and let the fact that you are rocking them in the gym while you do your thing speak for you. The time you carve out of your days in which to move your body and enjoy being physical is yours. Other people can either learn from watching you get your happily sweaty groove on, or not. Your teaching moment can simply consist of *your moment* . . . and your momentum. I guarantee you, it's one of the best teaching methods there is.

INCENDIARY ACT #6

CLAIM THE RIGHT TO BE UNATTRACTIVE (JUST LIKE ANYBODY ELSE)

You do not have to be attractive all the time—not by your own standards and not by anyone else's. Life is a come-as-you-are affair.

Just like everyone else in the world, you have the right to look like a normal human being doing normal human things. This is a perfectly acceptable state of affairs. You can put what you're doing ahead of what you look like anytime, sometimes, or all of the time.

You have the right to get sweaty and dirty. You have the right to sport visible hair on your legs, your armpits, and wherever else your body happens to grow it. You have the right to walk or run or bike or skate down the street in sweat-soaked workout gear with your head held high. You have the right to grimace and make faces when you're exerting yourself. You have the right to be unprimped and unperfumed and un-made-up.

You have the right to wear a ratty old T-shirt to exercise class. You have the right to wear Spandex. You have the right to have your hair plastered to your head with sweat or water or rain. You have the right to move in ways that mean that people are going to see your butt and your belly and your thighs and your upper arms and all the rest of it. You have the right to be flushed and red-faced and breathing hard.

You have the right to have cellulite where other people can see it. You have the right to have a belly where other people can see that, too, and the same goes for sagging breasts or missing breasts or scars or an insulin pump or whatever else you've got going on. You have the right to tie a bandanna around your head and not think about how it looks because it keeps the hair out of your eyes when you're concentrating. You have the right to not smile unless you feel like it, even if someone tells you to. You have the right to cause others to witness the sight of your completely unpedicured feet.

You have the right to not have to constantly manage how you look for other people's sake. You aren't here to decorate the world for other people. You're here to live in it for yourself, no matter what that looks like.

Finding and Creating Fat-Friendly Space to Move

Yes, Virginia, there is such a thing as accepting, friendly environments in which to move your body. It is totally possible for you, and other people like you, to have a place to move and play and enjoy the freedom of existing fully and happily in your body, no matter what its weight or size.

This may sound like something that only exists in dreams, but in actual fact, it is something that already exists in some places and that you can create for yourself if you don't happen to live in a place where there's already a fat-friendly venue for movement.

Searching online and in local information sources like newsweeklies, bulletin boards at community centers, and so on, is one way to find out what might be available to you locally. (Note: Because exercise classes and groups often come and go fairly rapidly, they are not listed in the Resource Guide in this book.) A good place to look specifically for them is *Kelly Bliss' Plus Size Yellow Pages*, online (which *is* in the Resource Guide). More importantly, ask around! You never know what connections your friends, coworkers, and neighbors will have. You may be pleasantly surprised to discover that there is someone local who has already put together a space, a class, or a fitness group explicitly for the purpose of providing a venue for people of a wide variety of sizes and shapes to move their bodies.

Do not be discouraged if you don't find any organization or group specifically labeled as "size-accepting" or "size-positive." Size-accepting spaces often exist without being labeled that way, not because they aren't size-accepting, but simply because no one has thought to label them that way. It's far from uniform, and you'll still have to do some sleuthing, but there are some trends in terms of where these spaces may be found:

- **Community centers.** Many people find that the more community- and family-oriented the exercise space, and the more inclusive the establishment is of people who don't fit the "young and athletic" stereotype of many commercial gyms, the more diverse and inclusive the establishment. My own experience has certainly borne this out: Jewish community centers, YMCAs, and municipal gyms and pools have been more diverse in terms of their clientele than most of the "health clubs" or "athletic clubs" I have spent time in. In general, such community spaces have featured people of a wide range of ages, sizes, abilities, and backgrounds, all taking advantage of the opportunity to enjoy moving their bodies.

- **Fitness classes for special populations.** "Special populations," in this sense, means "people whose physical needs differ in some way from the typical athletic body." In the fitness industry, "special populations" classes can include classes for pregnant women, for people who have medical issues such as heart disease or arthritis, for older exercisers, for people who have physical disabilities, and so on. It's also a category that can include classes specifically for fat exercisers. In the event that you can't find a class labeled as "plus-size fitness" and don't feel ready to face the jocks and jockettes in a regular class, you might try a class geared to people in some other "special populations" group. Some fat fitness fans have had good luck with classes geared toward people with arthritis or who have had joint replacement surgery. Such classes tend to include people of a wide range of body sizes and shapes. Additionally, everyone in the room has some sort of issue that presents a physical challenge, which can create some common ground. A tip: It's always polite to ask the instructor beforehand if it's okay if you sit in, especially if you're not a member of the class's target demographic.

- **Specialized skill venues.** This seems counterintuitive, but the more specialized the gym or class, and the more focused it is on the acquisition and development of particular skills and abilities, the less focused it may be on issues like weight, weight loss, or physical appearance. Boxing gyms, martial arts dojos, CrossFit training gyms, and circus-skill classes are all examples of venues for movement that can be quite size-accepting at the same time as they are physically intense. Because their focus is on what a person can *do* and not so much how they look or how much they weigh when they do it, these classes can be more comfortable for people of a wider range of sizes and shapes. Note that there are some specialized skill venues where this is *very much not the case*: disciplines like ballet, figure skating, gymnastics, and other activities that traditionally focus very much on body appearance and size are still unlikely to provide a size-accepting space.

What if you want to form your own size-accepting space for movement? Opening your own fat-friendly gym is probably beyond your means and your scope, though if it isn't, more power to you! For most people, the best place to start is simply getting together a handful of friends who are also interested in moving their bodies happily and in a supportive environment and doing things together. Maybe you'll set a time once a week to get together to go on a long walk. Perhaps you'll all go to a park with a pond where you can rent rowboats. Maybe you're bicycling enthusiasts, and you'll pick a different route to cycle together every week. Or maybe you'll all chip in to hire a fat-friendly fitness instructor to teach you a private class once a week, in the instructor's studio or perhaps in the home of one of your group of friends, should anyone have a space big enough. These are all ways you can start creating community and carving out some space where you can move your body in the company of people who are supportive, friendly, and sympathetic to your goals.

With a somewhat larger group of people, or more money to work with, you might be able to rent a space such as a church hall or community center activity room for regular activities or classes. It need not be the same sort of activity or class all the time. Perhaps you'd enjoy trying yoga lessons for six months, then decide that you all were curious to learn Afro-Caribbean dance for a while. Or you might add a second complementary activity to an ongoing one: members of a regular belly dance class might add an additional session of drumming every other week (drumming is very physical!).

You and your friends might even be drawn to move your bodies in performance groups. There have been, and continue to be, fat belly dance troupes, fat dance crews, fat burlesque groups, and even the delightfully named fat synchronized swimming groups the Padded Lilies and Aquaporko. Performance movement might not be your style, but if it is, it can be a radically life-affirming thing to do both for yourself and as a way of creating community and visibility.

One-off or occasional fat-positive movement events are also a great way of building community and creating space. Fat-acceptance activists in Portland, Oregon, developed a program called Chunky Dunk to make enjoyable, positive swimming more accessible to fat people. Chunky Dunk organizers "rent public pools and offer up a focused and intentional space where the natural diversity of human bodies is respected." The Chunky Dunk model would work just as well for renting a basketball court or a set of tennis courts, an ice-skating rink, or any other exercise-related facility.

When it comes to size-accepting exercise opportunities, the world is waiting for you to create your dreams. There are far more people out there who would love it if something active yet size-accepting existed in their areas than there are existing size-accepting fitness opportunities. Making the first move to create something like that in your area takes chutzpah! But some-one has to make the first move, and perhaps that someone can be you.

CHAPTER 3

What Am I Going to Do?

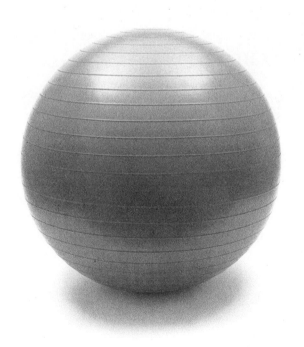

Now that you've decided that you want to belly up to the body-practice bar, and you've hashed through some of the emotional and psychological hurdles to getting there, it's time to get your move on. Finding out what kinds of activity suit you best can be a substantial project, because there are just so many different options, and physical activity is something you have to try in order to know how it feels. In this chapter you'll get a rundown on major genres of physical activity, their pros and cons, and just in case you need some motivation to experiment, even a list of one hundred things you can do with your body.

Stealth Exercise

Stealth exercise is the exercise you do that doesn't look like exercise. It is the exercise you get when you walk up a flight of stairs, when you stand up from a chair, when you walk your dog, when you fold the laundry, when you carry the groceries into the house, when you go out for a walk just because it's such a pretty day, when you get down on your hands and knees to chase after an earring that you dropped that rolled under the bureau.

Stealth exercise can, as the name suggests, be entirely invisible. For that very reason, it is one of the best bargains there is in the realm of movement and physical activity.

First of all, it's an excellent deal because it means you get to take credit for what you're already doing. Yes, I mean it—you absolutely do. And why shouldn't you? After all, your body doesn't care whether you move it in a gym or out of one, in a formal exercise setting or just going about your daily life. Movement is movement, and it's all good. If your body doesn't care, why should you? Especially if you're new to the idea of moving your body or feel really uncertain or uncomfortable with it, it can really help to give yourself some credit for the movement you're already engaging in. It can also be easier to stomach the idea of changing your body practice if that means just doing more of the same stuff you already do anyway.

· Second, stealth exercise is a bargain because it's unlikely to be perceived as "exercise" by potentially hostile onlookers. It's positively astonishing how going out for a walk dressed in exercise clothes and athletic shoes is an entirely different critter from going out to walk the dog wearing nothing particularly special. Hopping on your bicycle to go run your errands rarely pings anyone's radar (including your own) as a potentially reaction-causing "Awoogah! Awoogah! Fat person exercising off the starboard bow!" situation in the way that going for a lengthy ride on the nearest bike trail does. When you're moving your body in ways that people are likely to perceive as unremarkable day-to-day activities, they are simply less likely to cop an attitude. You're not doing anything out of the ordinary; you're just dropping off your library books, picking up a six-pack, walking your dog, and going to the post office, like you do.

Stealth exercise is also a great bargain because we ourselves can be just as easily fooled as anyone else. There's a very real sense in which walking the dog just doesn't feel the same as exercising. This is one of the reasons that doctors and fitness writers and other well-meaning people are constantly trying to convince people to do all those things like taking the stairs instead of the elevator or parking your car at the far end of the parking lot.

This, unfortunately, tends to produce a Catch-22 effect: when you start doing things to deliberately add more physical movement into your day, you tend to be self-conscious that you're doing it as exercise. Consciously adding movement into your daily routine is good in all kinds of ways . . . except for the part where you're so very aware that that's precisely what you're doing. Feeling self-conscious about it can be enough to make you not do it.

At the same time, for some people, stealth exercise can end up completely satisfying their needs for movement. Many of us in the United States do lead fairly sedentary lives, it's true, but the truth is that millions of people around the world—including plenty of Americans—get all the movement their bodies require just by doing a good variety of physical things in their daily lives. Most people around the world, after all, *don't* belong to gyms, don't go to exercise classes, and don't even so much as do workout videos at home. Their daily lives just include plenty of routine movement.

The key here is *routine*. If you'd like to get closer to getting all of your movement this way, it's critical to find a way to get past the self-consciousness to the place where moving your body more in a day-to-day way just feels normal. For some people, challenging themselves to add a new bit of day-to-day movement each week is a good strategy—perhaps the first week you decide you'll walk to the deli you like every day (that one that's a few blocks from work where you get your sandwich) instead of getting something from the coffee shop in the lobby of your building where you don't like the food as much anyway. Then the next week you can decide to take the stairs down when you're on your way to the deli instead of waiting for the elevator. And perhaps the week after that, you can take the stairs back up when you return. If you did something like this, you'd have added a fairly nice little chunk of movement into the middle of your workday. The fact that you'd also get some great sandwiches out of it just makes it better.

Obviously, this is a fairly specific suggestion and may not fit with your particular day-to-day experience. But there are always opportunities. Walk to the post office, the library, or the grocery store if the weather's nice. Get to your community event a little early and offer to help set up chairs. Stand up and walk around your workspace while you're on the phone instead of sitting still (I do this all the time; it also helps me make sure I don't get distracted by stuff happening on my computer screen while I'm supposed to be paying attention to whoever's on the phone!). Get up and walk to talk to a coworker in person instead of picking up the phone or sending email, a tactic that will also ensure that you get seen and recognized as a go-getter at work. If you're straightening up the house, walk each individual item back to its assigned spot in the house separately rather than gathering up a whole bunch of things at once and then dealing with them by the armful. Sure, it's not as efficient, but that's the point: you're using it as an opportunity to get more motion rather than expending less effort. Chances are good you can think of many other places in your day where this principle could be applied.

There are lots of ways that you can let more movement into your daily life, and the more often you do them, the less self-consciously aware you will be that you're doing so. That's when stealth movement really gets good: when you're moving around happily and not even thinking about it, just enjoying being active and interacting with the world.

Outdoors Versus Indoors

The decision of where you want to move your body can be a big one for the right-thinking fat girl. Indoor environments have a lot of things in their favor, to be sure. It doesn't rain on your head, the artificial light makes it easy to get your groove on before dawn or after dusk, and sometimes there's even air-conditioning in the summer and central heating in the winter. The surfaces underfoot tend to be more predictable and level, there is often a convenient bathroom nearby, and there's no need to worry about sunburn or poison ivy.

There are a huge array of indoor activities to try. Don't think you're limited to treadmills and aerobics classes! You can lift weights, try a spinning class, learn to swing dance, swing on a trapeze, take boxing lessons, do Pilates, shoot some hoops, develop your gymnastics skills, get your ping-pong game on, shoot some pool or play darts, and plenty of other things. Yoga! Exercise video games! Indoor rock-climbing gyms! And there are plenty of fun team sports that are often played indoors, too, if that's your thing, especially things like dodgeball, volleyball, kickball, and basketball.

Then again, there are plenty of reasons to love being outside: sunlight! fresh air! the wind in your hair and the allure of the open road, or bike path, or whatever it is, stretching out before you. Sure, there's the odd mosquito, and the terrain might get rough, but there are birds and flowers and trees and lakes and ponds, city streets to strut, window-shopping to be done, and let's not forget moonlit nights walking the beach. It's being out in the world, soaking it up, and there's a lot to like about that.

Going outdoors also offers you lots of possibilities in terms of activities you might enjoy. Walking, biking, hiking, running, and swimming are favorites for a reason, but don't forget about things like skiing, rowing, fishing, geocaching, golfing, playing Frisbee, snowshoeing, white-water rafting, and boogie boarding. There are also plenty of outdoor pursuits that may not sound much like "exercise" on the surface but that actually involve plenty of movement, like nature photography, bird-watching, and gardening. You can also combine outdoor movement and doing something for a good cause, too, with a charity walk or run, volunteering to plant trees or do a neighborhood cleanup, or that perennial favorite, helping a friend move by carrying boxes out to the moving van.

Indoors or outdoors, though, there are also some potential problems you have to negotiate.

First, there are other people. Unless you're on private land or at home alone, there's a good chance you'll encounter other people. In most indoor environments, the type of other people you will encounter is somewhat easier to anticipate than it is in the great outdoors. You get to know, for instance, what the clientele of a gym is like or who your classmates are at the dojo or the dance class. In these environments, too, there are written and unwritten rules that tend to get reinforced because people share space together.

In outdoor environments this is trickier. The more public the space—and you can't get much more public than walking down a street—the less you can guess at who else might be occupying it at the same time as you. People may be more prone to be rude or obnoxious in public spaces simply because they feel anonymous. But this is far from consistent. Some people report experiencing quite a lot of weight-related harassment in public spaces. Other people experience little or none. It can be hard to know why, and it can be hard to know what your own experience might turn out to be on any given day. The unpredictability of social interactions when exercising outdoors can make them less than appealing, particularly when you're feeling fragile or you're just starting out. But for many reasons, not least the simple fact that you're out in the world, practicing moving freely and happily in the world, outdoor movement is a wonderful thing when you're ready for it.

Second, there are physical safety issues. Indoor environments are simply more predictable, from a physical standpoint. There are fewer physical obstacles—broken pavement, tree roots, slippery patches, and so on—that could present a hazard. It's easier to control the level of intensity of your movement indoors, for instance, by adjusting the speed on a treadmill or picking up a different kettle bell, whereas the natural world throws hills and such things at you without so much as a by-your-leave, and if a big steep hill is between you and where you need to go, it's not as if you can just dial it down to something more amenable to your current fitness level. When you are indoors, unless you are alone, there's also a higher chance that there will be other people around who will notice and are likely to help if some mishap should befall you. Depending on your level of physical ability, your faith in your body and its abilities, and whatever medical issues you may have, this can be important.

Third, there's accessibility, both financial and physical. Access to indoor spaces that are not your own home and where you can engage in movement tends to cost money. You have to travel to and from them. One or both of these things may be an issue for you. Outdoor spaces, on the other hand, exist right outside your door, and you can walk out the door for free. Physical accessibility is variable, both indoors and outdoors. Assess your options, think creatively, and choose based on what fits your needs.

Solo Exercise

Moving your body all alone can be a glorious thing. There's no need to talk to anyone, and no one who is talking to you. No one is asking you questions or trying to engage you in conversation, asking you for input, requiring your attention. You can concentrate all your attention on moving your body and how it feels and not have to care a fig about much of anything else.

If you are a person who feels easily self-conscious or who worries a lot about other people's opinions, it can be a real blessing to have physical movement not also be a social event. But there are plenty of other reasons you might opt to get your bounce on by yourself. Perhaps you are one of those people who is constitutionally incapable of not getting competitive, and you don't really want to feel competitive about movement. Maybe you have a low tolerance for socializing and you'd just rather not have to have the additional pressure of being sociable on top of the movement thing. You might be a person who does an enormous amount of being sociable as part of your day-to-day life, working retail perhaps, and you just need a break from it. You might want solitude for strategic reasons, so that you can be fully conscious of how you're moving your body and can work on your form when you move. Or it could be that you are just one of those wacky individuals, not so unlike the author of this book, who finds that movement is a great time to meditate and just watch your thoughts flow.

There is often a lot of pressure put on us to make movement into a social event. For some people that's a really great idea. Most people enjoy doing things more if they're enjoying socializing while they do them. If that's true for you, and it helps motivate you to get your move on, then go ahead and make it as social as you want. But also bear in mind that there is no rule that says you have to.

Exercise Partnerships

You don't have to do it alone. That's the whole point of the exercise partnership. Partnerships forged for the sake of mutually increased movement and fitness can take many forms. There is the classic workout-buddy dynamic, where you and a friend or two get together regularly and do the same workout side by side. There are floating conglomerates of friends who meet up, in varying permutations of their members, for regular attendance at a particular exercise class. There are groups of people who band together intentionally to create size-accepting movement space or to pursue particular physical skills like dance or martial arts with like-minded folks. What is meant here by "exercise partnership" is any sort of sociable partnership you have with one or more other people that centers around physical activity.

For many people, exercise partnership is something that makes movement possible. Where they might've been overwhelmed with self-consciousness if they tried to go out for a walk or to a fitness class alone, suddenly it's not so bad if you have someone else along for the ride. Where they might've feared critical glares or commentary if they were by themselves, they might feel much stronger and more resilient knowing someone else is there with them. Where someone might have felt lonely or desperately wished for something to distract them from thinking too hard about the fact that they were exercising, having someone else there with you makes for good, and cheerfully distracting, company. It can simply be easier to motivate yourself to move if you know it's an excuse to hang out with people you like.

Not all forms of exercise partnership are the same. You can enjoy one but not the others, or you can like them all equally. You also aren't obligated to have an exercise partner for every kind of exercise you do. Having a partner with whom you do weight lifting does not mean you have to go bicycling together too. Having five people you like to go biking with doesn't mean you can't also have one person you religiously go swimming with. Be totally committed to walking five miles a day all alone, if that's what makes you feel good, and also totally open to driving across town to one particular dance studio because you know that's where you'll get to go to ballroom dance class with your old friend who always makes you laugh. Whatever works to make you feel happy, supported, and enthusiastic about moving your body is a correct answer to the question of "Should I have an exercise partner?"

Exercise partnerships can sometimes have a downside in the form of competitiveness. Being competitive is not a problem so long as a competitive dynamic is something you and your exercise partner(s) are looking for and can be open about. There are lots of people who manage to incorporate a healthy, friendly competition into their exercise partnerships and who really enjoy having someone not just to compare notes with but to compare performance with. If you both thrive on egging each other on or making bets about who will improve more or do better, then have at it and have fun. There's nothing like a competitive streak to add a little spice to your body practice and your experience of physical activity.

Then again, there's nothing like a competitive streak to make you angsty and tense, encourage you to feel like you are not good enough, and create a sense that unless you are able to compete (either with a partner or with the pros), you're just fooling yourself and you might as well not waste your time.

It can be hard to manage a strong competitive urge. It can easily get the better of us and drive us to push ourselves in foolish ways.

In the fitness world, there is a lot of talk about "personal bests," a way of formally describing competitions against ourselves, the push to do better than we did before, to lift more or go faster or work harder. It seems harmless enough to take your competitiveness and focus it only on yourself, but it's still possible to make yourself feel bad, injure yourself, or just overdo it in the hot pursuit of a personal best.

When other people are involved, it can get stickier still. Exercise partnerships can sometimes implode under the stress of unspoken but real competition or explode from the strain of competition even when it is open and aboveboard. Competitiveness is, after all, an emotion, something that we feel, and it gets bound tightly into feelings of worth and validity, competence and self-acceptance. Competition is dependent upon comparison and inequality. There is no competition when everyone is equal, after all, and relationships based in inequality have their pitfalls.

If you are a person with a strong competitive streak, it can be useful to find ways to let your competitiveness out to play without aiming it at anyone, except perhaps at yourself. The Internet has given us some surprisingly useful tools for this, particularly with participatory fitness communities like Fitocracy, which let you "level up" by engaging in and increasing various workouts and physical activities. Other online fitness communities like www.dailymile.com and www.livestrong.com provide social networking opportunities where you can, consensually and aboveboard, get competitive with friends or strangers, yet keep it at something of a remove. You may wish to experiment with these, if you are the type of person who benefits from a little friendly competition but wants to make sure that friendly—to yourself and to other people—is exactly the way it stays.

Group and Class Exercise

Finding the right exercise class is no small task. It takes some research, some time investment, and a bit of putting yourself out there.

What activities appeal to you? There are a lot of options out there, including (but definitely not limited to) yoga, aerobics, kickboxing, spinning, various kinds of dance, water aerobics, martial arts, core conditioning, and even specialized classes for moms-to-be, moms and babies, older exercisers, and people recovering from surgery.

Some of them will appeal to you or play to your strengths, and others will not. If you should come across a listing for a class in your area but aren't familiar with what it is—say, it's Zumba or urban rebounding or kettle bells—just look it up online where you can read about it and often watch videos of people doing it. If it looks like fun, and like something you might like to learn, off you go.

Before you sign up for a full series of classes, you'll want to talk to the instructor and sit in on a class. When you talk to the instructor, you should ask how he or she feels about having fat people in class. Fat fitness guru Kelly Bliss recommends just coming right out with it and asking "How do you feel about working with fat students?" Their reactions will often tell you everything you need to know; what you want to hear are neutral answers, not negative ones, and also not forced positive ones. Size-positive New York fitness instructor Rochelle Rice recommends the same and additionally suggests asking specifically whether the instructor is familiar with Health At Every Size (HAES) principles (see page 28).

You can ask whether the instructor is familiar with modifying movements for bigger bodies and is aware of some of the particular biomechanical needs of big exercisers that might require consideration, such as how to negotiate the moves when someone has a big belly or what to do when thick thighs make balance precarious if people try to keep their feet too close together. While you're talking, you can get a feel for whether or not this instructor seems like someone you would like to work with, and whether or not their priorities and interests seem to be in line with yours. Some people can handle it if an instructor puts focus on weight loss and calories and such during class; others can't. It's okay to have standards and boundaries about this and to choose a different instructor or class if one just doesn't seem like a good fit.

Make sure you sit in on a class before you sign up. You can't always tell how an instructor will be in the classroom on the basis of a one-on-one conversation. Just sit and observe from beginning to end, to see how the instructor works. You want to keep an eye on how the class flows. Does it seem balanced in terms of a good combination of movements and levels of difficulty for most of the participants, most of the time? Does the instructor watch for whether students are using correct form? Does she or he make helping individuals and answering questions a part of class? Do the people in the class seem to be happy to be there? Does the instructor speak compassionately and kindly to students when correcting or instructing them? Just as with anyone else, you can tell a lot about how comfortable you're likely to be with a fitness instructor by watching them interact with others.

When you actually start a group fitness class, you may find that the learning curve is steep. Particularly if you are joining an ongoing class, it may seem as if everyone else already knows all the moves and you are the only one flailing away valiantly yet still screwing it up.

Don't worry about this. Everyone else in the room, including the teacher, was a first-timer once too. Everyone there has been where you are. No one is born knowing how to sail through a yoga class or with an encyclopedic knowledge of every aerobics step. Do your best, and even if you haven't finished all the repetitions of an exercise by the time the class is moving on to the next, just move along with them. You may fall off the horse any number of times, but every time a new movement is introduced, you have a chance to get right back on. It can feel kind of hectic and harried to do this, but it also keeps you in the flow of the class and means that you don't end up feeling left out or like you're the lone straggler in the bunch. Just start anew with the next move and carry on from there.

It takes time to learn a new activity. Expect to attend several weeks of classes before you start to feel like you're getting the hang of it. The initial adjustment period can be a little rocky, so flail proudly (see page 84), keep yourself moving along with the class to the best of your ability, and in all likelihood, you too will soon be just another one of those people in the class who seems to know exactly what to do.

At Home in Front of Your TV

The idea of getting all the physical activity you need right at home, in front of your computer or your TV, is sort of the dream of fitness convenience. You don't have to deal with strangers, there aren't any locker rooms or parking lots, you can do it any time of day or night, and have I mentioned the part where it doesn't matter what you wear and you could even work out naked if you wanted? Sounds good, doesn't it? While it's never worked out well for me—I can work from home without problems and without getting distracted, but I've never been able to work *out* at home without getting sidetracked in 1,001 ways—many people swear by the privacy and convenience of home-based physical activity.

In theory, moving your body at home is not complicated. Simply clear some space and do whatever it is that you do. This might involve equipment or not. People often buy small equipment like hand weights and resistance bands for strength training at home. Those with more space and money may equip themselves with stationary bicycles and other fitness machines, perhaps even enough for a full-on home gym. But there are also plenty of people who do quite well with exercise that requires no equipment. Calisthenics are a surprisingly useful option for at-home workouts. Push-ups, sit-ups, crunches, jumping jacks, lunges, and all the other old gym-class faithfuls are classics for a good reason, and they certainly can get the job done.

But not everyone wants to be her own taskmaster. This is where video instruction and console game exercise come in. Video physical-fitness instruction has been around for a long time, since the days when famous fitness instructors like Bonnie Prudden and Jack LaLanne pioneered television exercise programming in the 1950s. These days, of course, we don't have to depend on broadcast TV for fitness instruction. When most people think of exercise videos now, it's DVDs or streaming video online. They're convenient, there are loads of options to choose from, and you can get a lot of variety in your workouts even if you have only a small library of videos. (They're also excellent if you like to talk back to the instructor, something that I, for one, have often been tempted to do. Unlike the person at the front of an actual fitness studio, the lady on the video will never know if you call her nasty names when she's urging you to do that particularly evil stretch.)

There are dozens, even hundreds, of good options in virtually every genre of movement you can think of, including tai chi, yoga, various forms of aerobics, various types of dance, strength training, and cardiovascular exercise. What's more, if you have Internet access, you can look up exercise video reviews before you buy, which can give you a better idea of what you're getting into.

Fitness videos are without question the easiest way to get access to fat-friendly exercise. Fat fitness guru Kelly Bliss has pioneered a website called www.phatmoves.com, which acts as a resource center and clearinghouse for size-accepting fitness, including a robust selection of fitness videos developed specifically for big bodies. Other options are available by search-ing "plus-size fitness" on sites like www.amazon.com. A list of highly recom-mended size-accepting fitness videos can be found in the Resource Guide of this book.

Console-game-based fitness options are a much newer genre of video-based fitness. The Nintendo Wii and the Xbox Kinect are currently the two leading systems, each featuring a large number of fitness titles. These, if you're in any way inclined toward video gaming, can be exactly the spoon-ful of sugar that gets the "medicine" of moving your body to go down the hatch with real pleasure and enthusiasm. With their attention focused on the game and achieving the various things the game demands so they can earn points, level up, and get their names on those leaderboards, many video-game exercisers don't really notice that they're exercising and end up spending more time than they expected moving their bodies just because they want to do well at the game. There's something kind of magical about anything that can make you forget that you're flapping your arms like a chicken or running in place, truth be told. When you follow the moves of video-game dancers on the screen, what you see always looks right, as opposed to seeing yourself in a dance-studio mirror, where somehow what you see always looks wrong. Even when the moves are silly, the games can be extremely engaging. Many people find that focusing on the gaming aspect lets them basically ignore the exercise part, and for some people, that's pre-cisely what they need.

Both of the major systems offer all of these perks. Both also have their limitations and their aggravations.

Although not all of the titles available for Wii Fit require you to use the balance-board controller, some do. The balance board has been criticized for confining the physical space the user can occupy when engaging in move-ment, which can feel unnatural sometimes. More problematic for many fat exercisers, the Wii Fit balance board also functions automatically as a scale and weighs the user on a regular basis whether she likes it or not. It has a weight cutoff of 330 pounds, which has been widely criticized for not being high enough. Another problem many people have with the Wii Fit system is its insistence on using weight change as its indicator of fitness progress. This is erroneous—weight does not correlate to fitness in any particularly telling way—and it can be psychologically hard to take for many people. If this sounds like it would be a problem for you, but you're still interested in getting your game on, look for titles that don't require the balance board, like EA Sports Active and Just Dance 2. Some games are balance-board optional, so look for that when you're shopping for games.

The Kinect, by contrast, uses cameras to track body motion rather than having the user interact with physical controllers, which means no non-consensual weigh-ins or weight-related bossiness. This also means that the user is able to occupy space more organically and freely. The Kinect sometimes seems to have difficulty tracking certain kinds of movements, which can depend on the size of the room and the version of the Kinect camera apparatus being used. (You can look this issue up on online forums if it is a concern.) Some people have also noted that the Kinect can be bad at accurately tracking the motions of large bodies. This can be frustrating when it happens, but it seems to be a bit unpredictable.

Both Wii Fit and Kinect Fitness libraries include many fitness titles and games. Some are better than others, and most have received at least some online reviews, so it is possible to get an idea of what you're getting into before you purchase or rent a game. As with any other genre of game, not everything will be to your particular tastes.

Fitness professionals are divided on whether console-game-based fitness is actually as productive, fitnesswise, as other means of engaging your body. Of course, much depends on what you choose to play: the WiiFit, for instance, has a meditation game in which the goal is to sit on the balance board with good balance and posture. This certainly has its physical benefits but isn't going to build a lot of strength or stamina. The various dance titles, including the popular "Dance Central" series for Kinect, on the other hand, will surely get your heart rate up. As tools for at-home fitness, console-game-based fitness systems are certainly interactive and enticing. Even at their least energetic, they are still going to engage more of your body than just your thumbs. If you're already given to gaming, or want the distraction that video-game exercise offers, though, they can be well worth the time and effort to get used to them. And hey, with all the dance titles available, you might even learn a few dance moves that you can bust out later on.

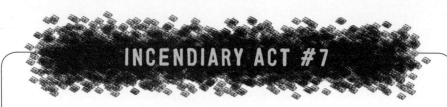

INCENDIARY ACT #7

FLAIL PROUDLY

In a perfect world, we'd all instantly be good at everything we tried. This is not that world. Sometimes we try things and discover we have a knack for them. Sometimes we have to work really hard to achieve anything like a basic level of proficiency. Sometimes we try something repeatedly and just when it feels like we're never going to get the hang of it, we do. Sometimes we flail a lot before we get anywhere.

Flailing proudly is hard, especially in front of other people. It can be really hard when it's obvious to others that you're struggling, trying but failing, or just not very good at something.

On the other hand, you don't get better if you don't try. And it's a lot more fun to try if you actually throw yourself into it and give it your all instead of pulling your punches and holding back because you're afraid you won't get it right. It's more fun because you're more invested. It's also more fun because if you *do* make some progress, or even get it completely right, you'll know what it really feels like to nail it, not just some dim shadow of what it might've felt like if you'd only committed yourself more.

With movement and exercise, flailing proudly is how you build strength and ability. Kittens go through weeks and months of being clumsy, uncoordinated little fuzzbutts before they are capable of the kinds of sophisticated coordinated movement that lets them be fluid and elegant and sly. We go through weeks and months of being slow and sluggish, of being stiff and inflexible, of not being able to hang on to the trapeze bar long enough to complete a full swing, before we find ourselves thinking, "Hey, I'm going pretty fast," touching our toes without noticing it, or flying through the air with the greatest of ease.

Flail proudly. Laugh as much as you can while you're at it: laughing helps you breathe more deeply and relax more, which tends to help your performance. Plus, let's face it, the whole process of learning new things can make even the most athletic among us look pretty goofy. A reassuring reminder of this is the Travel Channel program *Dhani Tackles the Globe*, in which pro football player Dhani Jones travels the world learning new sports—and often, even as a professional athlete, getting his butt soundly kicked. If a pro football player can flail proudly and laugh about it, so can you.

Team and Competitive Sports

There are an awful lot of people out there who believe that fat people simply aren't sporty. If fat folks were inclined toward sports, if they were the types to join recreational athletic teams or take part in amateur road races or get serious about tennis, the theory seems to run, they certainly wouldn't be fat.

Shows what they know. The truth is that there are plenty of fat folks who deeply dig being athletic in traditional, competitive sporty ways. I mean, have these naysayers ever actually *watched* pro football or caught a sumo match on ESPN? It beggars the imagination that people could possibly think there are no sporty, competitive fat athletes. There are fat tennis players and fat soccer hounds, fat softball mavens and fat field hockey fanatics. There are even fat marathoners and triathletes out there who routinely train at levels that would leave many thin fitness fans panting in the dust. Movement and body practice don't have to be limited to treadmill time or swimming laps or yoga class, after all. The world is your playground!

If competitive or team sports interest you, there is no reason in the world you should not pursue them and enjoy them to the fullest. It's my considered opinion that the more fat athletes take the plunge and participate in competitive and team sports, the more other fat athletes will see that it is possible and begin to follow suit. Many times, what keeps fat would-be sportswomen from becoming actual sportswomen is feeling like they'd be all alone. I thus heartily encourage you to get out there and play the game and see who else follows you onto the field.

Don't be daunted by the idea that you don't have what it takes to participate in a team sport or to compete with others. There are a lot of different levels at which you can take part. It's not all Ironman Triathlons and cutthroat tennis matches as intense as any Wimbledon match. Plenty of people play sports just for fun. Casual softball, soccer, and other team-sport leagues where you can just go out and knock a ball around are pretty easy to find in most places. Pickup games of Frisbee or basketball with your friends count, too. Even setting up croquet hoops on the front lawn during a family barbecue and playing a game with your nieces and nephews is a form of engaging in sports.

Getting into the nitty-gritty of serious athletic training for competitive or team sports is beyond the scope of this book. Different sports require different things, use different skills, and benefit from different approaches. There are many fine books, websites, and other resources out there dedicated to the specific training requirements of individual sports. The basic principles outlined in these pages, however, work as well for people who want to get involved in competitive and team sports as they do for anyone else. There is no sport for which a good strong baseline of general fitness is a liability! And there is no sport where trusting your body, trusting yourself as the authority on your body and your physical activity, keeping yourself active and moving, prioritizing your own comfort and health over arbitrary and external fitness standards, learning new skills, improving your physical condition as you go, and letting your pleasure in physical activity be the driving force behind your body practice will not help you excel. These things are just as important for the experienced marathon runner or the diehard swim-team stalwart as they are for someone just starting to think about how to make her life in her body better and more fun.

Personal Trainers and Coaches

The best way to think of a personal trainer is simply as a private instructor, someone who is to acquiring physical-activity skills what a piano teacher is to learning how to play piano. You can, naturally, learn physical-activity skills by experimentation and self-instruction just like you can learn to play the piano by ear and by playing around on the keys. You can self-teach with videos and books. But it can also be nice not to have to figure it all out for yourself.

Personal trainers are skilled professionals who have the background in movement plus the knowledge of how bodies work to help you find and learn the kinds of movement that will help you build your physical skills and improve your physical condition in the ways you want. Because you meet one-on-one, or sometimes in a small group, a trainer can provide you with individual feedback and specific information tailored to your needs. It tends to be very motivating, as well as sometimes terrifying, to meet with a personal trainer because you are being challenged to perform as an individual, with someone paying direct, immediate attention to what you do and how you do it.

Do be aware that personal trainers are not perfect. They are human beings with their own individual collections of prejudices and biases. There is no reason to expect that any individual personal trainer will have experience working with fat bodies. A trainer may or may not support the notion that a fat person might *not* be invested in weight loss as a major fitness goal. Personal trainers, by and large, are trained as part of an industry that is extremely committed to the thin, slender, athletic body ideal, so a trainer may assume that weight loss is an unquestioned good.

Don't forget that in addition to their fitness-industry training, personal trainers acquire their ideas about fitness and body practice from the same complicated, often toxic, sources that everyone else does. They may believe quite seriously that pain and suffering are a necessary part of physical activity. They may feel that fat bodies in particular deserve this as a kind of penance. They may have unrealistic ideas about what physical activity can accomplish in terms of creating particular body shapes, sizes, and appearances. They may be inclined to measure progress and success only in terms of pounds and inches rather than by more meaningful measures like functional fitness, blood oxygen level, or increases in strength and endurance. Worst of all, they may assume that thinness necessarily equals health and may push clients to lose weight at the genuine expense of their overall health and well-being.

What this means is that as an unapologetic fat girl who is a potential consumer of trainers' services, you must approach personal trainers with a good amount of skepticism and a big bag of questions.

First you'll want to be sure the basics are in place. You want to check a potential trainer's certification and make sure that she or he also has CPR and AED (external defibrillator) certification and perhaps also First Aid certification. Ask where the trainer works and what the fees are, including whether there is any extra fee to use the facility where the trainer works. Find out whether you will be expected to sign a contract for a set number of sessions and, if so, what the terms are and whether you can get your money back if you need to back out. Can you take a few sample sessions with the trainer before you commit to a contract? Will the trainer offer you some references to call to ask others about their experiences? Will you be alone with the trainer in the studio, or will other people be working there with other trainers at the same time? Ask!

Don't be afraid to ask specifically fat-related questions. You can, as fitness instructor Kelly Bliss suggests, ask "How much experience do you have with the unique biomechanics of big bodies?" and "When someone my size walks into your studio, do you form an idea of their fitness level based solely on their size or do you wait to see what happens when you fitness-test them?" The answers you're looking for are the conservative, technical ones, with information about mechanics and form, thorough evaluation, and testing. Rochelle Rice recommends that you come right out and ask the trainer if he or she will be comfortable working with you if you are not interested in losing weight, since some trainers have a very hard time letting go of that notion.

Here are some other questions you should ask any personal trainer you are interviewing.

- **What's your fitness philosophy?** A trainer should be able to tell you what his or her big-picture goals are in working with clients. She or he should be able to articulate whether the focus will be on body confidence, muscle building, strength, flexibility, weight loss, "body sculpting," or what-have-you.

- **How do you stay in shape? What is your own body practice like?** This will give you some insight into the kinds of priorities a trainer has for his or her own body, and hint at some of the priorities she or he may have in mind for clients. It will also suggest what kinds of movement the trainer likes best and may be most likely to use with clients.

- **Do you recommend supplements?** It's okay if a trainer has opinions about nutrition, but trainers are not nutritionists and giving clients detailed advice about what to eat or not eat or what supplements to take or not take is beyond their scope. If any trainer tries to sell you supplements or meal plans, pushes particular diets on you, or otherwise attempts to foist particular nutritional priorities on you (especially if they're selling them!), run, do not walk, in the opposite direction.

- **Are most of your clients long-term or short-term clients?** Unless your trainer is focused on very specific solutions, such as rehabilitative exercise, the ideal in the industry is for most trainer-client relationships to exist over the long haul. Certainly there are exceptions, but in general, if a trainer seems to have only short-term clients, be wary. It may be that she or he is burning out clients with inappropriate exercise, excessive demand, or poor interpersonal skills.

- **How did you get into personal training?** Asking for a little background information helps you get to know the trainer and also gives you some insight into how they think and feel about what they do and why they do it.

- **How many clients do you see in an average week?** This question will give you some idea about how booked your trainer is likely to be and how fresh he or she is likely to be when you have a session. Low numbers may indicate that someone is new in the field or that they are not very good at advertising, and not that they are bad at what they do. Many trainers do personal training as a part-time job and so keep their personal training hours deliberately low. The time to worry is when the number gets high: more than twenty-five to thirty clients a week means that your trainer is slammed and may be working by rote. If the trainer has more than thirty clients a week, you probably really don't want to be just one more cog in that assembly line.

There are also some questions that a personal trainer should be asking you. At a minimum, a trainer should ask you about three things:

1. **Your health and your health history.** A trainer should have you fill out a health history sheet for your file before your first session so that he or she can have all that information in one place. The trainer may ask you about injuries, joints and muscles, back problems, heart and breathing issues, and other things that might affect your physical activity or your ability to tolerate physical challenges.

2. **Your current activity level, what kinds of activities you currently do, and how often you do them.** A trainer should ask you about your current activities and levels. It's actually okay if the answer is "not much, not many, and not often" or even "I'm really not active at all, and I feel totally at sea, and while I want to change that, I need help and support and I'm scared." These are both answers your trainer should be comfortable with fielding. It's not okay for a trainer to dress you down for any

perceived failings in your fitness history, and it is really not okay for a trainer to mock or humiliate you. If this happens, *leave immediately*.

3. **Your goals for personal training.** Be very wary of being asked questions that may *sound* like "What are your goals?" but are not, such as "What is your goal weight?" The question "What are your goals?" is an open-ended one that can have all kinds of answers that may or may not have anything to do with your weight. Your goals may be general, like "I want to improve my overall condition and stamina" but this is also an opportunity for you to be more specific. You might say, "I'd like to work on my balance" or "I need to strengthen my lower back." It's also an opportunity for you to say what you really *don't* want, such as "I really hate exercise bicycles; I'd really like to avoid working on those." If changing your weight is one of your goals, feel free to talk about it, but beware of the tendency to make it into the only goal. Putting all your eggs into one basket is rarely a good idea no matter what, and when it comes to your body practice, too much focus on weight change can blind you to all the other things that are going on.

Functional Fitness

Here at Fat Girl's Guide HQ, we're deeply devoted to the notion of functional fitness. What functional fitness means is simple: improving the physical functioning you need to be able to do all the things you want to do in your everyday life.

For most of us, this is what's at the root of our desire to improve our body practice anyway. We want to be stronger and more flexible, have more energy and stamina, be less injury-prone and more physically resilient when we do get hurt or sick, and feel better physically in our own skins when we're going about our lives. Even for people who have specific skill-related or cosmetic goals for their body practice—let's say athletes who are in training for specific types of performance, or weight lifters who are attempting to increase the size of specific muscles—functional fitness is key. After all, almost everyone needs to be able to do everyday tasks like carrying groceries and moving our bodies from point A to point B, and that takes a certain amount of plain old physical capability.

The building blocks of functional fitness are very simple:

- **Stamina:** the ability to sustain physical effort or movement. This isn't just a matter of how long you can do a particular activity, but how comfortably. Stamina includes things like the ability of your heart and lungs to function happily over the long haul as you move your body, as well as everything else that contributes to your ability to keep moving over time.

- **Strength:** having bodily and specifically muscular power. Strength does not necessarily correlate with the size or visibility of muscles. We have many muscles that we cannot really see, such as the muscles that support the spine or hold your head up, whose strength is vital to feeling good and being functional in the world. Functional strength means whole-body strength, not just whether or not you can lift a barbell or "make a muscle" with your biceps.

- **Flexibility:** one's range of movement and ability to bend, stretch, and articulate the body and its parts. Being able to touch your toes is one demonstration of flexibility, but so is being able to reach around behind you and scratch between your own shoulder blades. Healthy flexibility doesn't mean contorting yourself like a circus acrobat, but rather possessing a full range of motion in all parts of your body.

- **Balance:** the ability to maintain physical stability. This means not falling over when you stand up! It is a combination of muscle strength (all that stability is generated by large and small muscles constantly adjusting your position) and proprioception (the unconscious awareness of the location and positioning of your body) working together to hold you upright when you sit, stand, go up and down stairs, ride a bicycle, and so on.

- **Coordination:** the ability to have two or more body parts and functions work together in harmony. Coordination encompasses a wide range of synergistic movement, whether it's being able to coordinate the use of two hands and two eyes to play the piano or coordinating all four limbs plus your head and breathing patterns to swim the front crawl . . . or even just coordinating your hand and arm to open a door and your legs to walk through the doorway.

Don't be put off by the technical-sounding phrase "functional fitness." It has become something of a buzzword in fitness training circles in the past few years, and people have come out with dozens of specialized techniques and exercises with a "functional-fitness" focus, but really it's not so specialized or complex as that might make it seem. Improving your functional fitness is easily done, requires no specialized equipment, and is something you can do both in everyday contexts and in workouts and other body-practice sessions. In fact, most specialized functional-fitness exercises are actually designed to imitate everyday movements and physical demands, for instance, the movements you'd make when lifting up a box and placing it on a shelf.

There are a number of different ways that you can approach functional fitness. They boil down to whether you would prefer the "buffet" approach, in which you incorporate a variety of different movement options that combine to hit all of the major building blocks of functional fitness, or the "one-pot meal" approach, in which you choose forms of movement that include all those components within single activities. You do not have to pick one or the other exclusively. Taking the buffet approach some days and the one-pot meal on others is perfectly fine. After all, the body is a generalist!

The Buffet Approach

The logic behind the "buffet" approach to functional fitness is based in the fact that our bodies are generalists, and they evolved to do many different things. Just as we don't need to include every single nutrient there is at every meal in order to stay healthy—because our bodies are good at getting the resources they need from what we eat over multiple meals and then storing and using them as needed—we don't actually need to include every single form of movement there is in every workout or activity session in order to enhance our overall functional fitness. Given a variety of types of movement throughout our days and weeks, so that all five of the major building blocks of functional fitness get some attention, our bodies will benefit in all those ways without our having to micromanage it.

No matter how much you love it, though, a balanced diet consists of more than just fried okra. We do have to organize our buffet plate a little bit for this approach to functional fitness to work well. Enjoying multiple kinds of movement is key. Consider mixing and matching from the following lists of activities that enhance your abilities in the five basic realms of functional fitness. Note that many types of movement have benefits in more than one area.

1. **Stamina:** walking, hiking, jogging, running, bicycling, swimming, water aerobics, rowing, skating, cross-country skiing, snowshoeing, elliptical trainer, aerobics, virtually all forms of dance, boxing, stair climbing, jumping rope, kickboxing, Zumba, yardwork/gardening, housework

2. **Strength:** swimming, Pilates, weight training, resistance band training, calisthenics, resistance exercises using body weight (sit-ups, pull-ups, push-ups), belly dance, rock climbing, most martial arts, yoga, kettlebells

3. **Flexibility:** yoga, tai chi (and other martial arts), gymnastics, Pilates, belly dance, modern or classical dance, stretching exercises, resistance band training, hula hooping

4. **Balance:** bicycling, skating, Swiss or "balance" ball exercises, skiing, yoga, martial arts, Pilates, virtually all forms of dance, balance or wobble board exercise, skateboarding, surfing, walking on sand/gravel/snow, pool- or water-walking

5. **Coordination:** racquet sports, volleyball, dodgeball, Frisbee, playing catch, basketball, yardwork/gardening, housework, jumping rope, boxing, aerobics, Zumba, Pilates

There are additional kinds of movement and movement education that can help you improve your movement skills and functional fitness. Many people who do not feel "at home" in their bodies, or who feel that they need help getting a handle on issues specific to flexibility, balance, and coordination find that taking some classes in the Feldenkrais Method or the Alexander technique are very helpful. These modes of movement education are based on the principle of helping people move their bodies more naturally and easily within the limitations of their particular bodies and their configuration. They can be exceptionally helpful for people who are new to movement, have movement limitations, are recovering from injury, or suffer from chronic pain.

The One-Pot Meal Approach

Finding a way to incorporate all the different realms of functional fitness into a single type of exercise or even a single exercise session can be tricky, but is not impossible. Some workout videos that are not marketed as "functional-fitness" workouts do a very good job of this: look for ones that incorporate resistance bands or hand weights (for strength training), aerobic exercise, and stretching or other flexibility exercise within the course of the workout. Other options for the one-pot meal approach include purpose-designed "functional-fitness" practices such as the high-intensity, athletically demanding CrossFit technique, which involves workouts with a wide range of exercises designed to challenge all parts of the body in all realms of functional fitness.

Another way to approach the one-pot meal of functional fitness is to simply engineer functional activities into your life that require aspects of all the major realms of functional fitness at a level that you find challenging and interesting. Heavy housecleaning and yardwork—the kind that requires a good mixture of lifting, bending, carrying, and walking—is genuinely excellent for functional fitness. Active child care often works well, too, or caring for animals, as anyone who has ever bathed either a three-year-old or an Airedale can attest.

Think about the kinds of everyday activities that left you feeling sore all over the next day the last time you did them, and you'll get a good idea of what kinds of everyday tasks might make good one-pot meal functional-fitness activities. By simply doing these kinds of activities in somewhat smaller doses, so that you don't end up quite so sore the next day, you can build up your stamina, strength, flexibility, balance, and coordination so that the next time you have to pull out all the stops to move house or go on a massive spring cleaning binge, you won't have to spend a week recuperating. That's the whole point of functional fitness . . . that you embark upon whatever activities you please and have the stamina, strength, flexibility, balance, and coordination to pull them off with pleasure and style.

101 THINGS YOU CAN DO
WITH YOUR BODY

1. Stretch, really stretch hard, when you yawn.

2. Bend at the waist and reach for the floor . . . even if you don't make it all the way.

3. Look behind you.

4. Kick! It's amazing how good just kicking can feel and how much aggression you can work out in the process. Take *that!*

5. Scratch your own back.

6. Pull your knees up toward your chest, as far as you can, while you're lying on your back and hold that pose for a few seconds.

7. Walk on your tiptoes.

8. Run! (There might be bears. You can't be too careful.)

9. Rip a cardboard box to shreds and then take the shreds out to the recycling bin.

10. Stroll, saunter, or promenade.

11. Have a pillow fight.

12. Skip! (It's so much fun, you won't care if you look goofy.)

13. Put on your sun hat, go out in the yard, and pull some weeds.

14. Put on your music and dance!

15. Scrub a floor the old-fashioned way.

16. Fidget.

17. Play Twister.

18. Dogpaddle.

19. Take a long, hot bath.

continued

20. Go ice skating.

21. Dig a hole. Moving dirt around is weirdly therapeutic.

22. Float.

23. Climb a tree.

24. Walk around the block.

25. Draw a hopscotch course and then hopscotch!

26. Go to a playground and swing on the swings.

27. Spin around in circles until you get dizzy.

28. Wade in a creek.

29. Go apple picking.

30. Do some of your laundry by hand.

31. Play catch.

32. Clean the bathtub.

33. Juggle—or have fun trying.

34. Change your perspective: hang upside-down from a jungle gym, a tree branch, or just over the side of your bed.

35. Play tug-of-war with a dog.

36. Take a walk on a beach.

37. Chase squirrels. (They could use the discipline, quite frankly.)

38. Row, row, row your boat.

39. Do the twist! The mashed potato! The Macarena! The funky chicken! Embarrass your kids!

40. Wash your car by hand.

41. Lie on the couch. (It may not be exercise, but it's still something you can do with your body.)

42. Roller-skate.

43. Take a toddler to the park.

44. Go inner tubing. Don't forget your sunscreen.

45. Rake leaves.

46. Haul out the trash.

47. Rearrange your room. (You were bored. Admit it.)

48. Learn a new dance move from YouTube videos.

49. Take a karate class.

50. Jump rope. Singing "Miss Mary Mac, Mac, Mac" is optional.

51. Play air guitar.

52. Take boxing lessons! Ka*POW!*

53. Go up the down escalator.

54. Rock climb.

55. Go birding.

56. Grab your boogie board and catch a wave.

57. Kiss. If this is not a whole-body exercise, keep trying.

58. Put a fresh coat of paint on something that needs one.

59. Go sightseeing on foot.

60. Plant a tree.

61. Get some friends to go to the park and play Red Rover or freeze tag. Yeah, you're a grown-up, and it's silly. That's the point.

62. Get some string and give your cat a workout.

63. Move your couch and find out what's under it.

64. Go to the farmers' market, wander around, and buy something that looks delicious.

65. Do the Time Warp! (Again!)

66. Swim underwater. How far can you go before you have to take a breath?

67. Play charades.

68. Learn to tango.

69. Fold the laundry.

70. Find a suitably grassy hill, lie down at the top, and roll all the way down. Climb back up and repeat. Whee!

continued

71. Play horseshoes.
72. Shuffle off to Buffalo.
73. Shine your shoes.
74. Go bowling.
75. Sing!
76. Give that special someone a lap dance.
77. Drop and give me twenty, soldier.
78. Bounce on a trampoline.
79. Give someone you like a backrub.
80. Throw a Frisbee around with a friend.
81. Fly a kite.
82. Climb the walls, if you must.
83. Croquet, anyone?
84. Make a blanket fort and hide out in it.
85. Blow bubbles.
86. Paint your toenails.
87. Go window-shopping. Stroll and browse and enjoy.
88. Take the time to cook yourself a meal you've been craving.
89. Build a sand castle.
90. Lift weights.
91. Collect all the stuff you've been meaning to put away properly and put it away properly.
92. Go to a nature preserve and walk a trail.
93. Learn to knit.
94. Refinish a piece of furniture.
95. Snowshoe.
96. Go to the playground and see if you can still do the monkey bars.

97. Make pasta from scratch and roll it out by hand.

98. Have really good sex, alone or with someone else.

99. Laugh.

100. Try a fun-looking exercise video from www.phatmoves.com.

101. Waterslide.

CHAPTER 4

Hit the Ground Running

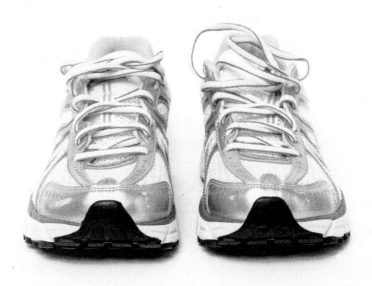

Ready to rock this out? Fantastic! Forewarned is forearmed, and in just a few pages you'll be ready to pick out a gym, face down the dreaded Locker-Room Thing, and even dive right into the pool (yes, even if you haven't been in one in years). Don't worry about what to wear, because we've got you covered from sports bras to shower shoes. From equipment weight limits to creative solutions to accessibility and fit problems, this section lets you break down whatever walls might stand between you and all the fabulous fitness you can handle.

The Unapologetic Fat-Girl Lowdown on Gyms

It's not just you, you know. There are actual reasons that you might not feel like you belong there when you walk into a gym. When you're not thin, male, and already immersed in the fitness scene, there are quite a few ways—none of them personal, few of them intentional—that most gyms are not built for people like you.

You'd think that gyms, of all the businesses out there, would have a vested interest in making sure that us fatties could get out there and break a sweat. It would seem to be part and parcel of the mission they claim to have. And yet here we are. Most gyms, most of the time, are more or less geared toward people who already fit the stereotypical profile of "people who go to the gym." Sure, lots of gym advertisements talk a good game about being places where everyone is welcome to come and "get off the couch," get fit, and engage in various sports and fitness activities. "New member" specials and "New Year, new you" advertisements suggest that they are open and accepting of people for whom going to the gym is a very new thing, and even for people for whom any sort of regular exercise is entirely new and unfamiliar.

In reality, most gyms, most of the time, are actually built and designed for people who are already relatively fit. Few have classes, equipment, or training intended for people who are well and truly newcomers to exercise, unless you're willing (and able) to shell out for a personal trainer to help get you up to speed. The equipment they have may not be appropriate for people who are beginning from a very basic fitness level.

Physically, gyms may or may not be places where your particular body will find a good physical fit. Most gyms are physically geared toward people of "average" body size, an issue that gets enforced by the standardized measurements used by manufacturers of most gym equipment from lockers to rowing machines to yoga mats. Gyms are also mostly designed and set up for use by able-bodied people. They're also, as I've heard many large-breasted women attempting to use weight machines complain, designed with men or small-busted women in mind. Gyms may or may not have equipment capable of handling people across a wide range of weights. Many gym-equipment manufacturers list weight limits that exclude some of the people who would really like to be able to use them, and gym management may or may not consider this to be an issue or try to preemptively provide a solution.

To some degree, this is only to be expected. Most businesses cater to the middle of the bell curve, because that's where there are the most people and thus the most money to be made. But in many ways, this is a shame. Everybody, and every body, deserves to be able to access places where they can move their bodies happily and healthily . . . including bodies that are far from already being fit, nowhere near "average" dimensions, have different physical abilities from the average, or simply weigh a lot.

When it comes to gyms, as with so many other things, we unapologetic fat girls have to take things into our own hands. However paradoxical it may be—and it is!—the fitness industry isn't always prepared to serve us and our needs. It's up to us to be informed consumers, to know what we're looking for, and to be assertive enough to make sure that we get what we want . . . or close enough for us to be able to do what we want and need to do as happily as possible.

What you're looking for in a gym is what everyone needs in a gym: a place where you can feel comfortable enough to work out, have access to the right equipment and instruction, and spend enough time to have the experiences you want. The list of questions in "Choosing a Gym" will help you ask the right questions when you're gym hunting, just as the "What Do You Think You're Doing?" and "What Do You Want to Do with Yourself?" sections earlier in the book (pages 17 and 21) helped you get some idea of what kind of experiences you're looking for and what sort of goals you have for your body practice.

Take these things seriously as you hunt for a gym to call home. It's easy to fall into the trap of thinking that one gym is just as good as the next, and, after all, a treadmill is a treadmill; how much difference can it make? You'd be surprised. Being at the right gym can make it not just bearable but sometimes actually pleasant to be there working out. Being at the wrong gym almost always means you just stop going.

Most regular gym-goers agree that you'll have a much better idea of what kind of gym is going to feed your meter and what kind simply isn't likely to get the job done after you've been going to the gym for a few years, just like you have a much better idea of what you want to look for in your next apartment or house after you've spent a while in your current one. It's always a learning process, but if you're proactive and ask the right questions, you can have a pretty good chance of finding a tolerably good fit from the start. Just the same, it's probably wisest not to get locked into long membership contracts right off the bat unless it's absolutely unavoidable. Occasionally, despite every effort, you'll join a gym and then discover some intractable problem. Even if you never switch gyms, you may as well do what you can to make switching gyms as easy on yourself as possible.

I'm not about to lie to you. It is easy to get intimidated when you're shopping for a gym and to feel that if you're not a "real athlete"—whatever *that* is—you don't have the right to have opinions about the gym, that any old gym should be good enough for the likes of you, that you don't deserve to have anything particularly special in terms of your gym because you're not in good shape, or not thin, or have a disability, or don't really know what you're doing in the gym to begin with.

Nonsense. If you're going to pay money to use a gym space, you have every right to make sure it's a place where you're going to want to actually do gym stuff. You should take a tour of any gym that you are considering and also ask for a guest pass so that you can come in on your own time to try out the facility to check it out at your leisure. Remember: In the United States and many other countries, businesses open to the public are legally obligated to make their facilities accessible to people with different abilities. It is not unreasonable to expect appropriate accommodations for your needs.

Don't be afraid to talk to people about their gyms. Talk to other people, especially other fat women you know, about what gyms they patronize and why they like them. Some fitness clubs and gyms specialize. They may feature racquet sport courts or ice-skating rinks or other specialty facilities, or have special fitness studios for things like spinning or aerial arts. Others are general purpose. Some gyms are devoted almost exclusively to fitness machines and other arrangements for solo, self-led exercise. Other gyms are heavy on the group fitness classes. Some gyms have a very heavy and intense agenda about weight loss or "body sculpting," while others are more aligned with a general fitness philosophy. And still others are extremely focused on building very specific skills, like rock climbing or boxing. Some gyms are single-sex, and others are coed. Some allow children, or have children's activities going on simultaneously, while others will be adults only. One gym is not necessarily the same as the next! Ask around, ask questions (a list follows!) and keep your eyes open.

Choosing a Gym: A Checklist

The following checklist will help you evaluate any new gym or fitness club you might be considering joining. Not all these issues will matter to everyone, and some will matter more to you than others. Your first impressions and gut feelings about a gym are at least as important as this checklist. Look around carefully and think critically, then take some time to check in with yourself before you sign on the dotted line.

Location and Hours

Don't assume you'll rearrange your life in order to get to the gym. Most people don't and won't, and why should they? A gym is a service business, and you are the customer. You are entitled to find one that fits with the life you have.

- Is the gym located in a place that is easy for you to get to? If it's hard for you to get there, you're not likely to get there often.

- Is the gym located near other places you regularly go, such as work, school, or your home? If it's easy for you to incorporate a gym trip into your daily rounds, you're much more likely to do so.

- Is the gym open during hours that fit your schedule and will let you be at least somewhat flexible about when you go?

Accessibility

Is the gym fully physically accessible to you, in terms of safety as well as usability? If not, don't be afraid to cross it off your list.

- Is the gym located in an area where you feel safe getting to and from the building?

- If applicable, does the gym have ample parking?

- Are there any indoor obstacles to your accessing all public parts of the building? Be on the lookout for any sort of obstacle that might affect your personal access to the facility such as turnstiles you can't easily fit through or toilet stalls that are too small for comfort.

- If child care is an issue for you, does your gym offer it? Or does it have children's activities available that your child or children can participate in while you are doing your thing? If so, is there an additional cost for this?

Social Factors

This category is hard to quantify but critically important, since if you don't feel comfortable with the social milieu at a gym, it can be miserable to be there. Your fellow gym-goers do not have to be your new best friends, but on the other hand, you aren't going to have a good physical experience if you're constantly having a conflict- or anxiety-ridden social one.

- When you visit the gym, do you get a sense of the clientele? Do they seem like people you'd get along with?

- Is the age range something that you are comfortable with? Sometimes people feel uncomfortable with a gym population that skews significantly younger or older than they are.

- Does the gym seem social, like a place where people are looking to hook up, or are the people there concentrating hard on their workouts? Is the vibe in the gym the kind of vibe you're looking for?

- Does the gym seem like a competitive space or a cooperative one? Is it a place where people appear to be acting like they're performing for others or a place where people mostly seem to be minding their own business?

- Do people smile back when you smile at them? Do you notice people chatting, or is it strictly a nose-to-the-grindstone kind of place? How does this feel to you?

- Is the gym's staff diverse in terms of sex/gender, ethnicity, body size/shape, dis/ability, age? Since you will be working with these people to get instruction and help with things, are you comfortable with the diversity, or lack thereof, in the staff?

Facilities and Equipment

The gym should have the kinds of equipment and facilities you want, and enough of them that you will be able to use them when you want and need them, in a safe, well-maintained, physically comfortable environment.

- Does the gym have the kinds of facilities and equipment you hope to use?

- Does the gym have a sufficient number of fitness machines to serve its population? There may be a wait for particularly popular machines during peak hours no matter how well equipped the gym. But gyms should make an effort to make sure they have enough machines of different types that this is not a common occurrence. Watch out for sign-up sheets: this is a sign that there are not enough machines and that people routinely must sign up ahead of time in order to make sure they get a chance to use a particular machine.

- Are instructions for machines clearly posted in easily visible places?
- Are staffers available to help you learn to use machines or to calibrate them correctly if you need help?
- Are there ample supplies of towels or wipes and disinfectant available for cleaning machines after use? Are they located conveniently? Do you see people using them?
- Do the machines appear to be well maintained and in good working order?
- Are temporarily out-of-order machines well identified with signs? Ask whether out-of-order machines are usually repaired quickly.
- Is there enough space for people to move around comfortably in work-out spaces and particularly in and among the fitness machines?
- Are the fitness machines you hope to use accessible to you? Do they have weight limits, and if so, are those suitable for your use? What alternatives are available to you if they aren't?
- If you use an assistive device(s) to move around, are there spaces where you can easily park your assistive device(s) within reach while you use machines? Will transfer from your assistive device(s) to fitness machines be problematic? If so, are staffers willing and able to help you?
- If there is a pool or hot tub, is it accessible? Are there steps or a ramp for easy and safe entry and exit?
- Are locker rooms, showers, changing areas, toilet/sink areas, and pool decks clean and in good repair?
- Are the benches in the changing areas or locker rooms comfortable and clean?
- Does the ventilation seem adequate? Does the heating or air-conditioning seem like it is kept at an appropriate level for the season and climate? (This seems trivial, but it can make a huge difference to your comfort and to your willingness to work out.)
- Are there lots of mirrors? If you are one of the many people who find it distracting or triggering to be constantly forced to observe yourself in mirrors, this is something to watch out for.

Classes and Instructors

At minimum, a gym should offer the kinds of classes you want to participate in, assuming you want to do group exercise at all. The instructors should be appropriately qualified and, optimally, also well disposed toward working with you and other people like you.

- Does the gym offer the kinds of classes you hope to take? Are they offered at times that will work for you?

- Is there an extra fee for classes? If so, how much is it? (Beware: These can add up fast if you are a fan of fitness classes.)

- Are specific instructors identified for specific classes (so that you would have the same instructor throughout), or do different instructors teach different class sessions?

- Will it be easy for you to meet or talk to instructors before taking their class(es)?

- Do you have to register for classes in advance, or are they available on a drop-in basis?

- What are class sizes typically like?

- Are gym staff courteous, friendly, and supportive?

- Are general gym staff trained to assist you in making the most of your gym time—helping you learn to use equipment, spotting you on a weight machine, answering questions?

- Does the gym have its own personal trainers on staff? Are they available for one-on-one sessions if desired?

- Is it possible for a member to bring in an outside personal trainer (i.e., a trainer who is not on the gym's staff)?

Cost

Gym memberships come at a wide range of price points. Sometimes it's hard to find one that has all the characteristics and equipment you want at a price point that you can afford, but at the same time, paying more than you can afford makes it easy to resent the gym. Cost and contractual obligations as a member are things that also affect your happiness with your gym.

- What is the joining fee?

- What is the monthly rate?

- Is there an additional annual membership fee? How much is it, and when is it due?

- Is membership "at will," that is, can you leave at any time, or are you locked into a contract of a certain length?

- How will you be billed for your membership, and what forms of payment do they accept?

Fat-Friendliness

This is likely to be the part of shopping for a gym where you will have to make the most compromises, because the nature of the fitness industry is that it assumes everyone who shows up is necessarily there, not to put too fine a point on it, because they believe fat is icky and they want to be thin. The notion that someone may want simply to be fitter, stronger, more flexible, and happier in her body, whatever the weight or size of that body may be, may be a new and unfamiliar idea to gym management and staff. Hold on tightly to this notion, though, for your sake and for theirs. Gym managers and staffers can't learn about something they never see or hear about. Show them and tell them by your example that you do, in fact, exist, and that caring about fitness and health and happy bodies means caring about *fitness and health and happy bodies*, not just about body size or weight or fat-to-muscle ratios.

- Do gym staff make assumptions about the reasons that you are interested in joining a gym (e.g., that you are joining because you want to lose weight)?

- Are gym staff open to and accepting of explanations for your interest in joining a gym that do not include or emphasize weight loss?

- Does the gym seem to be a welcoming environment for people of a variety of sizes, shapes, abilities, and fitness levels?

- Is there a strong focus on weight loss in the gym's various offerings and classes?

- Does the gym sell weight-loss products, foods, supplements, and the like? Is the gym making money by pushing diet products?

- Are there fat-shaming images or words in evidence in the gym's decoration, advertising, promotional materials, and so on? How many and how obtrusive are they? Would the management be willing to remove or change them for something more body loving and confidence building?
- Are members required to have an introductory set of measurements or weight recorded or to keep a chart that includes these figures?
- Are there dieting or weight-loss events held at the gym? If so, are you likely to be pressured to participate in them?
- Do gym staffers already seem aware that it is possible to improve health and to stay healthy at any body size? Do they seem open to learning about HAES principles?

The Locker-Room Thing

When we use the phrase "I felt naked" to mean that we felt vulnerable and defenseless, we aren't kidding. No wonder locker rooms can be so terrifying.

Let's be honest, there's not much to love about a locker room: all the unflattering lighting of a discount-store dressing room with none of the privacy, having to shove all your stuff into one of those dinky lockers, plus concern about whether you're likely to get athlete's foot from the floors, and the nagging little worry in the back of your head that anyone else who happens to be in the locker room with you at the time is looking at you and probably judging.

Lots of us fat girls have old, old baggage that we bring into the locker room with us. For some of us, locker rooms were the sites of some intense body shaming when we were at particularly vulnerable ages. For many of us, they were the places where we first saw our naked or nearly-naked fat bodies in direct comparison to thinner girls' bodies. Also, for some of us, the locker room was merely the agonizing overture to a humiliating and painful three-ring circus of gym-class ridicule, mockery, and sometimes outright abuse.

That's a lot to carry into a locker room. Alas, try as you might, you can't just cram it all into a locker and slam the door and leave it there. You have to deal with it one way or another.

Some people deal by simply not using locker rooms. They dress at home, go to the gym/pool, then come home to undress and shower or whatever they need to do.

But this can be inconvenient. Why should you have to be the one to deny yourself that convenience? Just because you're fat or old or funny-looking or whatever you are, it doesn't mean you don't have a right to some convenience in your life. After all, at the end of the day, a locker room is just a room with lockers in it. It's just a space. You have just as much right to exist uneventfully and usefully in that space as anyone. The question is . . . how?

The answer is planning and practicing.

First, get familiar with the locker room. Go in there fully clothed a few times without planning to use the locker room for anything. Make sure you know where things are. Where are the lockers? Where are the showers? Where are the toilets and sinks? Are there separate changing booths? Are there separate doors that lead to separate gym areas, like to the pool, to the basketball courts, to the main hallway, to the fitness studios?

While you're getting the lay of the land, you might want to consider what part(s) of the locker room seem like they'd be most comfortable. Some people prefer to be tucked in a corner. Others just want to be far away from the door. Depending on your needs, you might need to factor in physical accessibility issues. There's no rush. Take your time and get your bearings. You might be surprised how much of a difference it makes to your psychological comfort to have a bit of familiarity and know where things are.

Another part of planning for the locker room is packing your gym bag. Make sure you have everything you're going to want. Your lock is first on the list: you want a lock that is easy for you to use and that you can trust to be secure. Combination locks mean you don't have to fuss with a key, but putting a padlock key on a lanyard and hanging it around your neck while you work out means you don't have to memorize a combination.

Next up are gym socks, gym shoes, shorts or leggings, T-shirts or tank tops, your sports bra(s), swimsuit if you'll need it, shower shoes or flip-flops, toiletries, comb or brush, and whatever else you think you might need. I hate it when my hair gets in my face when I'm exercising, so I always need to pack a bandanna or scarf to wrap around my head. Some people find it reassuring and useful to take along a spare towel to put down on benches or chairs before sitting on them. I have also seen some women pack lightweight bathrobes to use in the locker room, for use when traveling between locker and shower (or sauna, hot tub, etc.). I've always thought it was classy, and besides, not all of us are of a size where wrapping a towel around yourself is going to get the job done. Having all your particulars handy makes the locker room easier to negotiate.

Once you've done this advance planning, it's time to use the locker room. Using a locker room doesn't have to mean getting totally naked. Some people find it easier to handle if it doesn't, especially at first. If you're nervous about being in the locker room, you might consider putting on your sports bra and your bike shorts (or your swimsuit, etc.) under your street clothes beforehand. Then you can strip down just to those, add the rest of your gym wear, and you're ready to go, without having to totally undress. You can also strategize what street clothes you wear into the locker room so that you don't have to remove all your street clothes to start putting on your gym clothes. You can, for instance, slip a pair of shorts on under-neath a skirt while you're still wearing the skirt, then take the skirt off after. You get the picture.

It is very much more the exception than the rule that anything bad happens in a locker room. Locker rooms are not, in actual fact, the secret clubhouses of the Effortlessly Thin Women's Fat-Lady Harassment Society. Sometimes people do get chatty in locker rooms, but in general it is the same kind of sociable conversation you'd hear in a doctor's waiting room or in line for movie tickets. You may encounter diet or weight-loss talk in a locker room, but it isn't necessarily aimed at you. (No, not even if that's what it feels like. Most gyms are well populated with people who are there primarily or even exclusively because they want to lose weight, after all. This presents issues, but they're not the same issues as being directly has-sled. Sometimes it really isn't about you.) On the whole, locker rooms are pretty businesslike places full of people who have things to do, like getting changed, perhaps showering or combing their hair, maybe putting on a little makeup before they head back out into the world.

For people who really get freaked out by the locker room, baby steps are sometimes necessary. Locker rooms usually don't seem so bad after you've spent a while just going into the locker room to use the toilets or to splash some cool water on your face when you're feeling flushed and overheated.

Occasionally you'll run into locker-room situations that are not as easily dealt with as others. It can be intimidating to find yourself the sole fat woman in a locker room that has just been overtaken by a svelte wave of spinning class devotees, leaving you suddenly feeling like a lonely rhino standing there in the middle of the Serengeti while a herd of gazelles surges past. Fortunately, rhinos are not known to be unduly impressed by gazelles, and you don't have to be either. Just remember that you're there for the same reason they are: to get your kit on and do what you came to do.

Locker rooms where you're changing alongside kids or teenagers can also be fraught. Children and adolescents can be particularly nasty and impolite just to impress one another. They are also often rowdy, loud, and leave a trail of chaos behind them, which is part of why many family fitness centers, YMCAs, and the like have separate locker rooms for the grown-ups. Use 'em if you've got 'em, I say. And always remember that you are the grown-up and have the right to insist that the management address the problem if there are unsupervised minors causing problems in a locker room.

So, the way you get comfy in the locker room is that you plan, you practice, and, when you need to, you psych yourself up. It's a public space, and you, my gorgeous unapologetic fat-girl comrade, are part of the public. The thing about public spaces is that in theory, we all get to share them. In reality, the people who get to share them are the people who show up and use them. Every time you show up and inhabit the space of the locker room, it becomes a little bit more yours, a little bit more a space where no one will be surprised to see you—or anyone else with a body that looks like yours. After a while you'll be able to approach a locker room as just a room with lockers in it, knowing that one of those lockers is yours.

Hitting the Showers

Showering at the gym is a lot like using the locker room at the gym, only more so. Why? Because you're naked! Naked, possibly somewhat blind because you're not wearing your glasses, and to make it all more complicated, you're touching your body, which calls attention to it in your own mind even when no one else can see you do it.

It can be complicated in other ways, too, even for the most physically unabashed of us. The physical setup of the shower space makes a big difference. Not all public showers are giant echoing rooms with multiple showerheads and no curtains or walls for privacy. In fact, most commercial gyms these days offer individual shower stalls, though the degree of privacy they offer can vary quite a bit. Sometimes these shower stalls are quite small; sometimes they are roomy. They vary enough that you'll have to take a look—you can't assume you know exactly what they'll be like.

For the sake of argument, let's assume that your locker-room shower is of reasonable proportions for your tastes and seems to offer enough privacy that you aren't too freaked out. How do you get from "not too freaked out" to actually being comfortable with taking a shower in a gym environment? The key is to negotiate the piece of the puzzle that lies between the locker and the part where you're standing there with the shampoo bottle in your hand.

Often, getting to and from the shower is actually the part where you feel most exposed. A cover-up of some sort is a really good solution to feeling like the trek from your locker is all too likely to be a Walk of Shame. It could be an oversized T-shirt, a sarong, a lightweight bathrobe, or anything that covers enough of your body to make you feel clothed enough to walk through the locker room. For some people a bath sheet or large towel brought from home may be sufficient coverage, but this doesn't work for everyone. (Never mind the dinky towels that some gyms provide with their towel service. Those are barely big enough to wrap around a wet head!)

Don't worry if this is not what other people in your locker room do. It may be that your particular locker room is one of those where most everyone wanders around naked. The whole "When in Rome. . ." thing doesn't apply everywhere. You are entitled to do what makes you comfortable. You have just as much right as anyone else to hit the showers and get cleaned up after a bit of good old-fashioned sweatiness, and whether you choose to do it at the gym or at home should be a question of convenience and personal preference, not one of fear or shame.

INCENDIARY ACT #8

KNOW THAT YOU'RE NOT ALONE

You are not the only person who struggles with the simultaneous desire to get up and move . . . and to sit on her butt. You are not the only person who gets resentful when someone who is "just concerned about your health" starts asking personal questions about your exercise habits. You are not the only person who often has to talk herself into just going out for a walk, much less actually kitting up and going to the gym. You are certainly not the only person who would gleefully deck the next person who self-righteously proclaims the results of her latest weight-loss campaign in public. You're nowhere near the only person who simultaneously wishes you could just be a "normal" weight and that people would lay off giving you crap about the weight you actually are. (You're also nowhere near the only person who also realizes that these are fundamentally the same wish: to not be harassed for your body size.)

You're not the only person who wishes she could magically be good at physical things, just so she wouldn't have to look like the stereotypical fat girl fumbling in front of all the jocks. You are so *very* not the only person who gets defensive about calling the shots regarding her own physical activity, and you're not the only person who actually ends up having to defend her choices because so many other people feel at liberty to criticize and comment.

You're not the only person who can be driven to hysteria by calorie counting, who would rather have a root canal than get on a scale in a public place, and who nevertheless finds it a source of deep joy to watch the miles mount up in her walking notebook. You're not the only person who wishes other people would, even once, just know to give her credit for all the hours she puts in at the gym or on the trail or in the pool. You're not the only one who gets frustrated when people assume that just because you're not thin, you've never broken a sweat in your life. You're not the only fat girl who finds great glee in surprising people with how strong you are or how much stamina you have or with the fact that you walk, run, swim, bike, and generally kick ass in a bunch of ways that always seems to shock people who assume that knowing you're fat means they know everything there is to know about you.

You are not alone with any of this. There is not a scrap of baggage about body weight and size and physical activity that you do not share with other people, not one—not the struggles, not the pleasures, not the ambivalence, not the frustration, not the joy, and definitely not the fear of criticism. It is all too easy to feel like you are the only one, to fall into the trap of believing that everyone else in the world is just more mature or more experienced or just plain better at doing the things you struggle with. Nothing could be further from the truth. Everyone else you meet is just trying their best, just like you are. It's okay. Do the best you can with what you have. You are not alone.

Play Pool

If I could, I would throw each and every fat girl who reads this book straight into the pool. Why? Because water is fantastic! It is soothing and centering and nurturing to be in water or even to be near it. There are reasons we like baths, soaks in hot tubs, wading in fountains, and even just taking showers. It's good for us.

For this reason, if nothing else, it is well worth finding ways to get your fat, fabulous, ferocious self into the pool, lake, river, pond, or swimming hole at least occasionally. Mind you, moving your body in water also has a lot of fitness-specific benefits to recommend it. It's an awesome way to get low or even no-impact exercise. It's easy on your joints. It makes it almost impossible to notice whether you're sweating, which is an enormous bonus if you don't like to sweat. Water simultaneously provides support, in the form of buoyancy, and resistance, in the form of friction between the water and your body and the density of the water itself. You can safely and relatively easily do things in water (for example, handstands and somersaults) that could be difficult and possibly hazardous to do on land.

You don't have to know how to swim to enjoy exercising in water. Any form of water exercise, even if it doesn't feel terribly strenuous, lets you easily and efficiently build strength throughout your body. Walking in waist-deep water, for instance, is a great workout and feels fantastic. You can't go as fast as you can on land because you have to push through the water, and that's precisely what makes it both fun and challenging. Water aerobics are fun and splashy and goofy, you hardly notice that you're sweating, and they can give you a startlingly thorough workout.

All this, plus it's relaxing and good for you to be in the water. It promotes lymphatic drainage and good circulation, improves mood, and is excellent therapy for arthritis and other musculoskeletal problems. So why aren't you swimming right this minute?

If it's because you're afraid of being seen in a swimsuit, you're not alone. If you're like many fat girls, you may not even *own* a swimsuit because it's just been so long since you were willing to be seen in one.

I am pleased to inform you that this situation can be remedied.

A swimsuit is just a garment you wear in the water, something that's made to get wet and to still fit relatively well when it is. There is no actual reason that it has to look like a traditional tank suit or bikini or cute one-piece, with or without a darling little skirt. You can, of course, find all those things for sale in plus sizes. But if you prefer more coverage, there are also board shorts, tankini tops, and numerous other types of swimwear that offer far more coverage. Rashguards are basically T-shirts made of swimsuit fabric, originally devised for surfers, which give you all the coverage (and sun protection) of a T-shirt without sagging and bagging when they're wet or billowing away from your body when you're in the water. Aquatards are leotards made for water workouts, with shorts- or capri-length legs; some aquatards have sleeves as well. You can get swim separates, tops and skirts (with built-in briefs beneath) in a variety of lengths and degrees of coverage. The options are a lot more varied than they used to be!

This does not mean that you are going to find the magic swimsuit that makes you look skinny. This is because you're not skinny, and that is perfectly okay. You can still find a swimsuit that is comfortable and wearable. Given that it is possible to assemble swimwear that covers you up to the neck, down to the elbows, and all the way to the knees, you are in no danger of being forced to expose intimate bits of your naked self to the world. If you're able to leave the house in something less than an ankle-length down-filled parka, you will be able to find swimwear that will give you almost as much physical coverage as anything you'd wear on the street, and in sizes at least up to a 6X. (See the Resource Guide.)

If you avoid the pool because you are worried about being able to get in and out of the water, you're not alone there either. One of the joys of being in the water is that buoyancy counteracts a lot of the effects of gravity. It's just so easy to move around in the water! But getting back out onto dry land can be hard, as you stop having the advantages of the buoyancy and begin to feel the full weight of your body again. Even if you are merely walking back up out of a lake or the sea through water that gets shallower and shallower, it can be a rude surprise to feel your body getting heavier and heavier as you go. Having to deal with this as you attempt to haul yourself up a pool ladder that may be narrower than your body makes it that much worse. As for hoisting yourself up over the edge of the pool with just your arms and legs, well, not even all slender people can manage that.

If you have any worry about your ability to get in and out of the pool, look for pools that have ramps or stairs. Many pools have these types of entrances these days for disability access reasons, another way in which good accessible design ends up being good for everyone.

Safety and Weight Limits

How can you tell what sports or fitness equipment is safe for fat people to use? The fear of having equipment fail or, worse still, break while you are using it, is an insidious one. No one wants to be the person who flattens the bike tire or breaks the elliptical trainer. No one wants to have to actually *be* the horrible, humiliating punch line to a tasteless fat joke. It's enough to get you to just not take the risk. But not only is it a sad loss of potentially useful and pleasurable stuff in your life if you avoid any sort of sports or fitness equipment, it may also be unnecessary.

The simple fact is that there are an awful lot of people who are worrying about weight limits who have no need to whatsoever, because their weight simply does not exceed them. Most run-of-the-mill fitness equipment is officially rated by its manufacturers to be suitable for users up to at least 300 to 350 pounds, with some fitness machines officially rated safe for user weights up to 500 pounds. Some pieces of equipment, including ones you might not expect, are rated even higher than that. The standard-issue, major-manufacturer exercise ball I keep in my office for impromptu back-stretching sessions is rated up to 300 kilograms, or 661 pounds . . . and there are heavy-duty versions that are rated to even higher weights.

What most people don't realize is that a weight limit is not, in fact, an indicator of the point where the object in question self-destructs into a billion tiny little pieces under the almighty onslaught of too much fatness. It's merely an indicator of the point where the manufacturer will no longer allow itself to be held legally responsible for the item suffering a failure to perform. It's fair to think of a published weight limit as the manufacturer's way of saying, "Well, we know for a fact that it'll perform properly with *less than this* amount of weight on it. Whether it'll perform properly with more? We aren't sayin', *just in case it doesn't*, because we don't want to get into trouble if we're wrong."

In other words, it can be useful to know what weight limits are on specific pieces of equipment, particularly if you're going to the expense of buying and maintaining one for yourself. But those limits are definitely not gospel. I have watched lots of people of lots of sizes of fat use lots of different exercise equipment in my time, and I have yet to see anything break or fail in a dramatic way, or at least not in any way I haven't seen the same machines fail when they were being used by thinner exercisers.

If you want to know the weight limit for a particular piece of equipment, these numbers are usually given somewhere in the user manual. It may take a little digging to find the information, but it's typically in there somewhere. If it isn't, you should be able to get it by calling or emailing the manufacturer.

Just remember that a weight limit is not a magic boundary that cannot be crossed or Bad Things Happen. It's just a statement about known and tested performance, and a limitation of liability.

Comfort and Ergonomics

Fitness equipment designed for people with middle-of-the-bell-curve bodies is not always comfortable or orthopedically sound for anyone else. Fat athletes may find that handlebars, pedals, and footrests are too closely spaced for comfort. Settings to adjust the height or angle of a seat or backrest may not allow enough adjustment for the user to achieve proper form. In some cases where the user is expected to fit into an enclosed or semienclosed space, there simply may not be enough room.

There are too many possible situations in which fitness equipment might present problems of fit or ergonomics to list them all here. There are so many different types of fitness equipment and so many bodies of a wide range of shapes and sizes that you could imagine a nearly infinite variety of potential issues. No matter what the problem is, however, you can make a reasonable attempt at addressing it by asking the following questions:

- What is the nature of the fit problem? What part(s) of the equipment are not fitting well and in what way? How is it affecting your body? How would it have to change in order for you to be comfortable using the equipment?

- Is there an alternative piece of equipment that will perform the same function but with fewer fit problems? Sometimes, for example, a gym will have more than one model of elliptical trainer, treadmill, or stationary bicycle, and one will be a better fit than another. They are not all made on the same plan, and the differences in usability can be quite startling. If you have trouble with weight machines, you may be able to do similar exercises with free weights (which have additional fitness advantages anyhow, since they require you to use more strength to control the weight and maintain your form). It is worth trying whatever's there. You may be pleasantly surprised.

- If there is no alternative piece of equipment available, is there an easy potential fix for the one that is available? Can a handlebar be moved or removed, a pedal extender added between the crank arm and the pedal of a bicycle or stationary bike, or a wider footrest attached (temporarily or permanently) to the existing one? Can the seat back be taken off or laid flat?

Sometimes it can take creative problem solving to address a comfort or ergonomics issue with a piece of fitness equipment. Even in gyms, equipment modifications are not necessarily out of the question. Talk to your gym manager and see what they can do to help. Some people have been pleasantly surprised to find that gym managers have even had items on hand— pedal extenders for stationary bicycles, for instance—that have helped to address their fit problems simply and immediately.

Yes, asking for help and accommodation can feel embarrassing. Remember that it is the *equipment* that does not fit. It is totally legitimate to say,

"Hey, this machine doesn't fit my body" because it's true. Machines and other inanimate objects should conform to the needs of human beings, not the other way around.

A Fitness-Equipment Shopping Note

If you are shopping for a piece of fitness equipment for yourself, first do your homework. Find out about any relevant weight limits and read reviews online. For items that are mechanical, call around to a few area fitness-equipment repair places and ask them what they recommend as being most reliable and sturdiest: they are in the position to know what breaks down least.

When you're ready to buy, remember that unless you are prepared to deal with returning potentially very large and unwieldy items, it is a good idea to try them in person first. Brick-and-mortar fitness and equipment stores are the best place for this, even if you later end up buying your equipment from online stores. Get on that bicycle and, after you've had the staffer adjust it for you, take it for a ride. Try out the exercise ball; see how it feels. Climb on that aerobics step and make sure it doesn't feel like it bends under your foot when you jump on it. Get into that kayak and pretend to paddle for a few minutes and see how things shake down. If the pedals on that elliptical trainer seem like they're too close together, ask the salesperson if there's a model with a wider foot base and see if that feels any better.

You'd try on a new pair of shoes before you bought them, wouldn't you? You'd walk around the store in them, test them out, and see how they felt and whether it seemed like they pinched or gapped, right? Fit is no less important here. And considering how much fitness equipment can cost, it only makes sense to make sure you are investing your money in something that fits you properly.

Dressing for It

I'm going to say this once to get it over with: yes, you can do your physical activity in the oldest, schlubbiest, ugliest, most ill-fitting ratty clothes you own, but you shouldn't.

Even if you never leave the house, it's hard to feel good about what you're doing when you're wearing your most unspeakable outfit. It's hard to feel like movement is something you should take seriously if your sole priority in terms of getting dressed for it is to put on clothes no longer capable of being ruined.

This is not to say that you must wear only pristine color-coordinated carefully chosen workout clothes specially bought for the purpose. Nor is it to suggest that you must immediately go out and spend money you don't have on exercise clothes you'll feel weird about wearing.

It is to say that perhaps you could stand to work out while wearing the *second* rattiest clothes you own, just on principle.

Ideally, the clothes you pick for physical activity should have most of the same attributes as the clothes you pick for any other purpose. They should fit you properly, they should be well made and durable, and you should like their appearance well enough to wear them regularly. I'm going to address each of these issues in turn.

Proper Fit

For a whole lot of reasons, the clothes you wear to move in should fit you properly. Skintight garments are sometimes appropriate, if they've got the stretch to make sure they move with you and fit well enough that they don't bunch, ride up, or otherwise make a nuisance of themselves. Oversized items, on the other hand, tend to get in the way. They flap and bag and sag, especially when they get wet with sweat. They can get in the way when you're moving and can even get tangled in equipment. It's also much harder for you or anyone else to assess your form if you can't actually see your own body for the vast swathes of fabric wafting in the breeze.

If you are prone to buying clothes in a larger size than you really need on the theory that if your clothes are baggy—or "flowy" or whatever you want to call it—then people are less likely to notice that you're fat, go right ahead and do that, just not for your physical activity wardrobe. A baggy T-shirt is not a magical invisibility cloak. No one will be fooled. You might as well wear something that fits you properly.

Your gym clothes, ideally, will skim your body without being clingy, unless it's something that is supposed to be tight. The shoulder seams will hit at your actual shoulder, and the arm holes will be big enough for comfort but not so big that the side of your bra is on display. Pants or shorts will let you move comfortably, including bending easily at the waist and knees. Sweatpants are sometimes a good idea and sometimes not so good, depending both on how baggy they are, how warm they are, and whether you're exercising in the cold. Getting overheated during movement is something to avoid, so lighter-weight pants, leggings, or shorts are often a better idea unless you're exercising outdoors in cool or cold weather.

You'll need clothes that suit the conditions you'll be in. Outdoor exercisers will likely require more gear to cope with temperature extremes, inclement weather, and so on, while indoor exercisers really don't need to worry about that stuff.

Quality

Exercise clothes take a beating. They are subject to a lot of friction and stress and sweat. Because they get sweaty, you will want to wash them frequently. It is rarely a bad bet to buy the best-quality clothing you can afford, but this is even more true in the case of exercise clothes. Look for substantial fabrics, solid stitching, and things that seem as though they will hold up well. Do not purchase anything with complicated care instructions. Carving out the time for physical activity is difficult enough; why should taking care of your gym clothes be difficult too?

Do not give in to the temptation to buy the lightest-weight fabrics you can find on the theory that you're going to be hot when you are moving your body. Light-weight fabrics are somewhat cooler, yes, but they also tend to wear out faster and give you much less protection from chafing and other abrasions.

What fibers you choose is a personal decision, but be warned that cotton, a common choice for gym clothes, is not always optimal: it gets wet and stays wet when you sweat in it. This can be a liability for long or intense workouts, particularly if it's hot or if you have sensitive skin. Many of the new "technical" and "wicking" fabrics do a much better job of keeping moisture away from your skin.

Appearance

The most important quality in athletic clothes is not their appearance but their performance. They need to do a particular job for you, and as a result, they may not be as fashion-forward as you might ideally wish. Still, within the parameters of getting that job done, you should definitely choose workout wear that makes you smile when you catch a glimpse of yourself in the mirror.

No, a T-shirt and bike shorts is not the most imaginative ensemble, and that's just fine. No one is going to accuse you of looking like you just stepped off the catwalk when you roll out for a bike ride with your big, goofy, and totally essential helmet on your head, and that's absolutely okay, because a brain injury isn't exactly this season's finest fashion accessory either.

Workout clothes may never be what you feel you look best in. You can still choose colors, prints, and styles you like. There are a lot more cute movement-friendly clothes available in plus sizes now than there were even ten years ago, so don't despair until you've done some Internet window-shopping (see the Resource Guide for places to start). You don't have to wear gray sweats or stick to white T-shirts or be condemned to an eternity in those little tennis socks with the pompoms on the heels . . . unless you like that sort of thing. You can jazz up your workout outfits with colorful scarves to hold your hair out of your eyes, fun socks or sweatbands, and garments with clever sayings emblazoned on them. Personally, I long for a pair of gym shorts with "WIDE LOAD" appliquéd across the butt and a T-shirt that says "I came here to lift weights and kick ass, and I just finished lifting weights." Now *that* would be an unapologetic fat girl gym outfit to be reckoned with, don't you think?

The Well-Shod Fathlete

It is unfortunately true that good, properly supportive, durable footwear for physical activity tends to be expensive. On the other hand, these are your actual feet we are talking about, the ones you will be walking on, and kicking butt with, for the rest of your life. Treating them as well as you can manage isn't just a good idea—it's an important part of making your body practice something that will be productive and sustainable for years to come.

If you haven't been fitted for athletic shoes, it's worth doing. Stores that cater to runners are a very good place to get fitted for athletic shoes. Their staffers are trained to measure feet accurately and to ask the right questions about what kind of support your particular feet might need. Do your feet tend to roll outward? Inward? Do you have flat feet or high arches or a narrow heel? All of these things and more can make a huge difference in the kind of support and protection your feet need to be consistently comfortable and protected while you are active.

Shoes are constructed based on forms called "lasts" that approximate the shape of a human foot. Not all lasts are shaped the same way, which is why not all types of shoes, or even all models of shoes within a single brand, will fit your foot equally well. Specialty shoe shops whose staff members are knowledgeable about which types of shoes tend to fit which types of feet are familiar with the quirks of each last, and they can help you figure out which shoe manufacturers and which specific lines are most likely to suit your needs.

Many people benefit from an athletic shoe that offers some motion control. This helps reduce any tendency one might have for the strike path of the foot to veer toward the outside edge of the foot (toward the pinky toe) or toward the inside edge of the foot (toward the big toe). To assess the amount of motion control a particular shoe offers, first squeeze the heel of the body of the shoe, where the bottom of your own heel would be if you were wearing it. It should be very stiff and not flexible. Next, hold the heel of the shoe in one hand and the toe in another and see if you can twist the sole of the shoe at all. The sole should resist twisting but have a little bit of give.

As a general rule, athletic shoes designed for cross-training are the best general-purpose athletic shoe. They offer a level of cushioning, support, and stability that is intended to work for a variety of activities, including running, walking, court sports like tennis or basketball, and fitness classes. However, should you do a lot of one specific activity, like playing squash, running, walking, or hiking, you may wish to consider looking into a shoe that is expressly constructed to help your feet cope with the demands of that specific activity. Running shoes, for instance, tend to be lightweight and often are made with breathable materials to help keep feet comfortable during high-intensity activity, but they don't always have the durability of walking shoes or cross-trainers. Hiking shoes or boots are quite heavy and protective with very thick and rugged soles for better traction on rough or slick terrain, but you wouldn't want to go for a run in them.

Some shoe brands that have a good reputation among big-bodied and wide-footed athletes include New Balance, Brooks, Saucony, and Propét.

People who do a lot of water exercise, especially water aerobics, may wish to look into special water shoes. Pool surfaces are often intentionally gritty or grooved, which is great for traction but abrasive on bare feet. Support issues are not a real concern here in the same way they are on dry land, but making sure that the shoe fits snugly enough and can be secured effectively to your foot is important, since you don't want your shoes coming off and floating away in the middle of a pool session.

A Word About Bras

The thing about moving your whole body is that your whole body moves. It's science: Newton's First Law of Motion states that an object in motion tends to remain in motion unless some other force is exerted upon it. Isaac Newton never actually wrote about breasts and their tendency to get jolted, jostled, and jiggled when women exercise, but he certainly would've understood the physics.

For small-busted women this is not typically too much of a problem. Smaller breasts are more easily strapped down with a typical sports bra and require less structural support to stop them from moving when you don't want them to. Sports bras that fit smaller cup sizes are relatively easy to find, too, even if your band size is large.

Larger-breasted women, on the other hand, have a harder time. Bigger breasts have more mass and thus more momentum once they are in motion: it simply takes more to control that motion. Normal sports bras may just not be big enough to fit properly, and even if they are big enough, they may not be sturdy enough to let you avoid discomfort. For women with very large busts or very large band sizes, it can be hard to find any bra in your size, let alone genuinely suitable athletic bras.

What to do? Some women find that doubling up and wearing two standard sports bras, one over the other, helps. Some women have success with buying a sports bra a size smaller than they would normally wear, simply for the sake of the compression, but this can get uncomfortable. Many larger-breasted women find that sports bras constructed with individual cups are more supportive than the less structured "shelf bra" sports bras. (Sports bras with actual cups also cut down on the "uniboob" or Breastloaf Phenomenon.)

If you have trouble finding a good sports bra (or a good bra in general), it is a great idea to find an old-fashioned bra shop and go in and get yourself fitted. Many lingerie shops are equipped at least to measure you and help you figure out what size you require, even if they may not stock your size. You can always get measured and then take the information elsewhere, including to online vendors.

A somewhat more expensive option, but a very good one indeed, is to have your sports bras custom-made to your measurements. Enell, a highly regarded maker of sports bras for large-busted women, offers this service (see the Resource Guide). Their bras have a reputation for very good motion control and are also reputed to wear very well, making the investment worthwhile.

Coping with the Belly Flop

The Belly Flop is related to the breast momentum issue. Just as breast-shaped objects in motion tend to stay in motion, so do belly-shaped ones. Experiencing uncomfortable and sometimes embarrassing belly flopping and jiggling can certainly put a cramp in your athletic style, especially when you are running or engaging in other high-impact activities.

The solutions are imperfect at best; there are no formal athletic under-garments for women that are designed to control the motion of a fat belly. People do, however, use various types of stretchy, tight-fitting garments to help hold things in place: leotards, unitards, and one-piece bathing suits can help. Personally, while I am not given to wearing "foundation garments" like girdles or other "body shapers" under my street clothes, I have found that the Spanx line of body shapers can be a boon if you are endowed with a belly big enough to be subject to the laws of physics in ways that get annoying. Spanx makes several variations on the unitard, all reasonably durable and with a high degree of compression. It feels a little strange wearing what is basically a girdle under gym clothes, but it does help keep the belly flop at bay and is worth a try if you enjoy high-impact activity.

CHAPTER 5

Action and Reaction

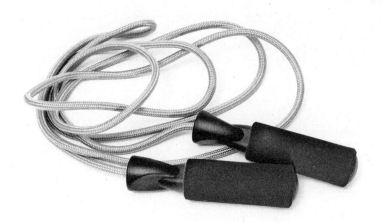

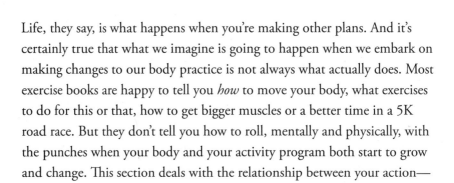

Life, they say, is what happens when you're making other plans. And it's certainly true that what we imagine is going to happen when we embark on making changes to our body practice is not always what actually does. Most exercise books are happy to tell you *how* to move your body, what exercises to do for this or that, how to get bigger muscles or a better time in a 5K road race. But they don't tell you how to roll, mentally and physically, with the punches when your body and your activity program both start to grow and change. This section deals with the relationship between your action—your body practice and your movement in the world—and your reactions, as well as ways to learn from and grow with your experience of being active in your body.

The Long Haul

In the beginning, exercise is easy. Not physically easy, perhaps, but it's easy to motivate yourself. It's easy to go do this fun new interesting challenging thing because, well, it's fun and new and interesting and challenging.

In the beginning, you really notice when exercise makes you feel good. You notice feeling stronger, feeling more energetic. Your body is bubbling and humming in a new way because you're doing a new thing, and it tends to make you want to get more of the good stuff.

In the beginning, you're in a honeymoon period. Everything is shiny, and even the things that hurt do so in that good, rewarding, "That's right—that's what happens when you're an asskicker" sort of way. .

And then one day you realize that it doesn't feel that way anymore. It's become humdrum and ordinary and it's not really all that fun. Oh, you might still feel better if you do it, but not in the fizzy-champagne sort of way, more just an absence-of-feeling-cruddy way, which, let's be honest, is nowhere near as engaging. You find that you have to remind yourself to go get some exercise. You may even have to strong-arm yourself. Or you may just not do it at all because it's not fun anymore, and anything you have to force yourself to do soon becomes something you dread, and we all know where that leads.

If any of this describes what you've been through with exercise, or what you're going through right now, congratulations: you have reached the dreaded Long-Haul Slump.

In most long-term relationships, including your relationship with your body practice, something like this is eventually going to happen. Familiarity may not necessarily breed actual contempt, but it sure isn't as much fun as novelty. When things become routine, they can become dull. It gets easy to lose interest. Especially if the thing in question is not something that has a lot of positive associations in the first place and may not feel like it has a lot of built-in immediate rewards, well, it isn't really shocking that you might be wandering around like a Method actor muttering "But what's my motivation?"

What you're dealing with isn't abnormal, in other words, and it's not unexpected. But it also doesn't have to derail you.

It helps to know what's going on when this happens. Part of it is the psychological stuff, the way a new thing becomes routine, the way that changes in how you feel and what your body can do become the new normal. But part of it is also physical and physiological.

When you first begin a new body practice, your body rises to the challenge. Improvement in your physical capabilities happens when your body responds to you placing increased demands on it. Often it can respond quite quickly at first. Eventually, though, your body will hit a level of physical ability where the curve gets steep, and it takes either a much longer time, a significantly increased effort, or both to push your abilities to the next level. The same old routines, activities, and intensities just can't give you the same bang for your buck because your body has gotten to the point where those are old hat: your body is in cruising mode.

When you get to this point in your body practice, there are several things you can do that will help you keep on practicing more happily and willingly.

First, you can stop worrying about it and just keep doing what you've been doing. The Long-Haul Slump happens to everyone, but there's a secret: it'll pass.

Yes, it really will. (I promise.) If you keep at it and keep going back to the gym or the park or the pool or wherever, and you keep moving your body and doing your body-practice thing, eventually you'll swing back around. Things will get fun again. You'll find new enthusiasm.

People experience this differently. Some people get short but relatively frequent bursts of having everything feel wonderful and fun, amongst the stretches of ho-hum. Or you may be one of those people who periodically gets a whole new honeymoon experience that lasts weeks or months at a stretch, perhaps because you've changed your routine or tried out a new activity, or maybe just because your body hits a particularly good stride with an old routine. Different people have different patterns, but most people find that if they can just get through the dull bits, eventually the shiny parts reassert themselves and you get all excited about it again.

Second, you don't have to let it run the show. The Long-Haul Slump is mostly just a silly brain trick. You're bigger than it is. Many people find that once they get going, moving their bodies provides enough momentum that they manage the rest of their workout just fine.

And don't forget: if you've embraced movement in your life, you can embrace this, and there are good reasons that you should. The Long-Haul Slump is a sign that you've actually gotten comfortable, that this whole moving-your-body thing is becoming second nature, that you've actually gotten used to it both physically and psychologically. Especially if you've always been shy about getting in the game, physically speaking, getting to the Long-Haul Slump is actually an enormous and important step. Look at you: you've been moving your body often enough for long enough that you're bored with the same old same old. Talk about a cloud with a silver lining. Did you ever think you would get that far and get yourself moving often enough, for a long enough time, that it'd become routine? That's why I meant the "congratulations" part when, earlier in this section, I said,

"Congratulations: you have reached the dreaded Long-Haul Slump." You'll experience some, perhaps all, of the different modes in which these plateaus can arrive and come through the other side just fine. In the meantime, job well done.

Play, Work, Meditation, and Vitamin Pills

Over the long haul, your relationship to moving your body will change. Your feelings about it will shift and mutate. You won't always feel the same about it as you do now, or as you will in six months. Sometimes it will be easy to get yourself to exercise. Other times it will be like pulling teeth . . . from a marble statue. There will be many states in between. This is all normal and natural and utterly to be expected. Rare is the human being who always feels exactly the same way about something all the time!

There are four major dynamics that tend to come up for people with regard to physical activity. Each one has its own challenges in terms of motivation, and each one affords its own unique opportunities for developing your body practice. I call these four dynamics play, work, meditation, and vitamin pills.

Play

Play is straightforward. It is the dynamic where moving your body feels playful, exciting, and fun. Sometimes this is the proverbial honeymoon period after someone has just begun a new body practice, and everything is still shiny and new. Sometimes it's because you've brought some other positive new thing into your movement life, like a new exercise class you love or maybe even just a new pair of gym shoes. (I know I'm not the only person who delights in the springy bouncy sensation of a brand-new pair of trainers!) Sometimes it just happens—you go to get some exercise one day and you just feel fantastic and everything you do seems like fun.

It's easy to motivate yourself when you're in the play phase. It can even be easy to motivate yourself to work extraordinarily hard when this dynamic is in force because you're enjoying yourself, and pushing yourself becomes a delightful game. Beware of the tendency to overdo it! Overuse injuries are tremendously common when people are in the play phase. Unfortunately, this can lead to a nasty cycle in which you get all excited, overdo it terribly, spend painful time recovering, then feel as if you just don't trust or like being physically active because every time you do it, you end up hurting yourself. You don't go back to it for a long time . . . until the next time you get swept up in the play dynamic and overdo it and you hurt yourself all over again.

It's also very easy, in the play phase, to succumb to overinflated expectations. When everything feels exciting and invigorating and like you can do anything, it's easy to fall into the trap of thinking that physical activity will always feel that way, that you are a natural-born athlete after all, and that every magical result you have ever hoped for from physical activity is going to manifest in your life within minutes. As with overdoing it physically and sustaining overuse injuries, this too can end badly, and in much the same sort of cycle of hurt and frustration just described that leads to abandoning physical activity altogether, at least for a while.

The key to the play dynamic is to enjoy it and take advantage of what it has to offer, but not to take it too seriously or presume that it isn't going to change. Euphoria is a lot of fun. But it is also a gift. Don't take it for granted, and you should be just fine. The take-home message of the play dynamic is this: *if it seems too good to be true, it probably is, so enjoy it to the hilt but keep your eyes open and your wits about you.*

Work

Work is also straightforward. This is the dynamic where physical activity feels, well, a bit like punching the clock. It's not fun or spontaneous. But just as with showing up at your place of employment, showing up to the work of your body practice is a necessary part of getting the job done. This is the essence of the long haul of any body practice, as discussed in the previous section: just keeping on keeping on.

When I am deep in a work phase with my own physical activity and body practice, I sometimes end up doing my entire workout in ten-minute intervals. The trick starts with getting my gym kit on and telling myself, "Okay, you only have to do ten minutes." Having gotten to the end of one ten-minute chunk, I think to myself "Well, I'm not miserable, this isn't awful, I could do another ten minutes . . . but I still get to quit after that if I want to." And off I go for another ten minutes, and usually another ten after that, and so on. Six of those little "just ten minutes" and amazingly enough, I've done a whole hour of physical activity, even though I never committed to more than ten minutes of work. And here's a confession: if I'm really cranky and I really feel like moving my body is a giant laborious pain in the ass, I'll even do it in five-minute increments. (Hey, sometimes ten minutes seems like a *lot*.)

Every so often, it's okay to let yourself off the hook. Just like with your job, every once in a while, if you really need the mental health day, you just take it. You can do the same with your body practice. It's totally fine and in fact really healthy to remind yourself that no, you aren't chained to anything, that you really are calling the shots, and that the flip side of the discipline it takes to go to work every day and get the job done is the freedom to occasionally decide that you don't have to do it *right now*. The take-home message of the work dynamic is this: *work takes discipline, in the form of showing up and putting in the time to get the job done, but bear in mind that this is a decision you make about a job you wanted for a reason, and it matters that you have a choice here.*

Meditation

Meditation is an interesting dynamic to find yourself in with regard to physical activity. This is the dynamic some people arrive at where physical activity becomes a contemplative area of their lives, a realm that is in some ways profoundly separate and different from the rest of what they do. In some cases, meditation is part and parcel of the type of physical activity the person engages in: martial arts and yoga tend to have a culture of meditation that is an inherent and intentional aspect of the physical practice. But you do not have to be a yogini or a martial artist to find yourself experiencing a meditation dynamic in your body practice. Many people end up feeling this way simply by dint of repetition, doing the same physical things at regular intervals over and over again. Because of this tendency, the meditation phase sometimes flows out of the work phase.

As with the play dynamic, motivating yourself to get off that chair and move your body can be relatively easy when you're experiencing physical activity as a mode of relaxing, positive-feeling downtime. Unlike the play dynamic, though, feeling the meditative groove of long-term repetition is unlikely to get you to push yourself too much. The meditation phase is all about being able to relax into what you're doing, to enjoy the predictability, and to reap the benefits of movement without feeling overtaxed.

This is actually just fine in a lot of ways. There's nothing the matter, physically or psychologically, with reaching a point where you're comfortable and simply maintaining that. There's no truth to the notion that unless you are constantly pushing yourself, you're somehow failing to accomplish what you should be in terms of fitness. Once your body arrives at a level where it is comfortable, it actually tends to do very well with simply maintaining that level.

Actively meditating while you move can be part of this. Some people like to concentrate on their breathing, while others like to silently repeat an affirmation or mantra that is meaningful to them. Sometimes I like to use a heart-rate monitor and concentrate on keeping my heart rate very steady, using the biofeedback of the heart-rate monitor as a place to focus my attention. I have talked to people who like to pray their way through exercise sessions, and to other people for whom just paying attention to the rhythmic motions of their bodies is enough to let their minds empty of pretty much everything else. Experiment to see what works best for you.

The real problem with the meditation dynamic is that it can be boring. This may or may not be a problem for you. (See "What's So Bad About Boredom?" on page 37.) The other issue that crops up with the meditation phase is that, like the others, it does not always last, and having it fall apart can be a little jarring. Forewarned is forearmed. The take-home message of the meditation dynamic is this: *your body and mind like the reassurance of knowing they are getting what they need, and gratifying those needs doesn't have to be either dramatic or exciting to feel good and get the job done; it's okay to have your body practice simply not be a big deal.*

Vitamin Pills

A "vitamin pill" is what I call the physical-activity dynamic where your relationship with movement centers around a specific desired result. Often the result is something related to health, like reducing blood pressure, improving insulin sensitivity, strengthening joints, recovering from injury or surgery, or regulating mood. You know you are in the vitamin-pill dynamic when the thing that motivates you to move your body is the awareness of that payoff. It becomes a transaction: you want the results; you swallow the pill.

The vitamin-pill phase of your movement relationship can sometimes be triggering for people who have a complicated emotional relationship with physical activity. It can strengthen your commitment to your body practice to realize just how strong a reaction your body has to physical activity, but this realization may also leave you resentful that it is in fact the case. You may simultaneously feel fortunate to be able to affect your own body in such a hands-on way (one that gives you so much power and control) and feel helpless in the face of the fact that now it seems like your body is demanding something of you that you may not always feel like or be up to providing for it.

Particularly when you're fat, having it become very plain to you that your body truly does want and need the exercise you've been giving it can bring up a lot of baggage about other people's expectations regarding fat people and exercise. It can feel like you're being forced to buy in to the old tired notion that fat people have a moral obligation to exercise because they're fat, or that everything that is wrong with you is because you're fat and you don't exercise enough. Worse, you may feel as though everyone who ever made you feel bad about your size was right—it really *was* as simple as getting more exercise . . . except that it isn't, and you know it. Movement helps, sure. But it helps everyone. You have the same kind of physiological responses to physical activity as everyone else. It's not special or different or more or less moral or what-have-you because you're fat.

Over the long haul, the vitamin-pill dynamic tends to intersect a lot with the work dynamic, although sometimes, pleasantly enough, it also intersects with the meditation dynamic. The take-home message of the vitamin-pill dynamic is this: *sometimes physical activity can simply be a transaction you engage in with yourself for pragmatic reasons, a way to give your body what it needs so that it has the best possible chance of doing the things you need it to do.*

The 80 Percent Rule

I want you to forget everything you've ever heard about how you have to "give it your all" for exercise to do any good. Erase from your memory phrases like "no pain, no gain" and "go for the burn" and "maxing out." Feel free to set fire to the idea that unless you're "giving 110 percent" you might as well just stay in bed. None of it is true, and all of it can exhaust or even hurt you. Instead of 110 percent or even 100 percent, set your sights on 80 percent. It's much more reasonable, rational, and, effective over the long haul.

Here's why: Within tolerances that vary from person to person, the body will adjust to the demands you put on it. Exercise instructors call this the "principle of overload." Lift a lot of boxes every day and you get stronger; ride your bike a mile or two a day and you get faster and better at biking. That's roughly how becoming more physically fit and competent works.

But it doesn't happen all at once. Even if you push yourself to the absolute utmost of your physical ability every day, you will not magically be a professional athlete by the end of the month, or even by the end of the year. Nor will you turn into some kind of superhero just because you work so hard that every muscle screams. The body doesn't work that way. The body can only get stronger or more limber as quickly as it can, and it can only do so as part of a cycle that includes rest, repair, and regrowth. The same is true with regard to competence and skill. Your brain and nerves and muscles can only learn new skills, or refine old ones, as fast as they are capable of learning.

Pushing too hard often results in overstraining your muscles, ligaments, and joints, which are then more easily injured because they're already strained. It's also a pretty reliable recipe for frustrating yourself because you're pushing so hard and still not, somehow, managing to magically change things as quickly as you'd prefer.

Like it or not, this body-practice thing takes time. That's okay. Time is actually on your side simply because you're always going to have a body, so you have plenty of time to work on it. What you need is a rule of thumb that lets you push, but push in a way that doesn't become counterproductive.

Giving it 80 percent—not 100 percent—creates this useful balance. Working at 80 percent of whatever you feel like your peak effort is at any given time, you will get enough of a challenge that things stay interesting and productive without so much of a challenge that you hurt yourself. It will provide enough of a push that your strength and stamina and flexibility will improve by adjusting to the demand without pushing you so much that you get destabilized or overstressed.

There are a couple of ways to figure out where your 80 percent is at any given time. One way is to periodically test yourself by pushing as hard as you can for a very short time, being careful to back off the instant you feel like you're hitting your limit or feeling any pain. From there you can either calculate or estimate where your 80 percent falls.

For instance, you might gradually ramp up the weights on a lat pulldown until you can no longer complete the exercise, then use the last weight that you *could* handle—the weight where you "max out"— as your 100 percent mark. From there, you can easily subtract 20 percent, rounding up or down to the nearest convenient weight available. So if you maxed out at eighty pounds, then eighty pounds is your 100 percent. Divide eighty by five to get 20 percent, which in this case is sixteen. Subtract that 20 percent from your 100 percent and voila: 80 percent, or in this example, sixty-four pounds. Because gym weights usually come in five-pound increments, you'd probably want to round that up to sixty-five. But if sixty-five pounds proves too heavy for you to do all the reps you wanted to do, you could always round it down to sixty pounds instead. So 80 percent is a rough goal, not an immutable law.

If you are using a treadmill and discover that 4.3 miles an hour is your maximum rate, 4.3 mph becomes your 100 percent for the time being. Since 20 percent of 4.3 is about 0.86, that brings your 80 percent to 3.44 mph. If 3.4 mph feels a little too slow, round it up to 3.5 mph instead, and if 3.5 mph feels like it's a little fast, round it down.

You can also do a version of this with only a watch or clock. Count the number of movements you make in ten seconds of peak effort—how many steps you take or strokes you make or whatever—and adjust to 80 percent of that. If you make 12 strokes with your kayak paddle in ten seconds at your peak, then 80 percent is about 9.6 strokes, which you can safely round up to 10 . . . or down to 9 if that feels better.

It's a good idea to check on your 100 percent and adjust your 80 percent about once a month. You should also check your 100 percent and adjust your 80 percent any time you feel like your 80 percent is becoming consistently not the right kind of challenge—either too easy or too hard.

This brings us to the other method for determining your 80 percent, namely, the subjective estimate. It is less precise but sometimes more usable, particularly when you're moving in ways that don't lend themselves to easy numerical measurement. It also involves pushing yourself as hard as you can for a very short time, then backing off until you feel like you're somewhere around 80 percent of that maximum. If you're accustomed to using the 1-to-10 scale for evaluating your effort discussed in "Getting the Right Feedback" (page 29), what you're looking for here is something around a 7 or an 8 on that subjective scale. This is useful when you're doing an activity where there just aren't speedometers or clocks, or the activity is simply not the kind of thing where it makes sense to measure things in terms of some objective quantity like pounds or miles per hour. It's okay to trust yourself to know what the intensity of your effort is.

The 80 percent rule often works best with a combination of these two approaches to finding your 80 percent. What your 80 percent is on any given day will probably change. People find that their physical capacity fluctuates depending on all kinds of factors, including hormonal cycles and stress and how much sleep you've been getting. You are not obligated to stick to your mathematical 80 percent if you're having a bad day, and right now, what should be 80 percent feels more like 300 percent. You are also not obligated to stick to your mathematical 80 percent if you're having an awesome day and what normally feels like 80 percent feels like it's only about 50 percent. What feels like 80 percent *right now* is perfectly fine. You are completely entitled to trust your own judgment about what that is. Remember that bodies, and their reactions, change for various reasons. As you build your workouts—and as you do them—your subjective experience of your effort may change. Respect the feedback you're getting and adjust accordingly. Pushing in sustainable ways is helpful. Pushing in unsustainable ways isn't.

Building a Workout

If you're ready to get moving, you're ready to learn a little about structuring a session of physical activity. There are lots of different ways to go about it, and none of them are wrong. Some of them work better for certain purposes than others, but ultimately, the most important factor in terms of how you put together your movement is whether or not you feel comfortable and if your body seems to hum along nicely throughout the session and you feel good afterward.

The classic way to structure a session of physical activity is to follow the format of warm-up followed by a period of intense activity followed by a cool-down period. Let's say you plan to move your body for a total of a half an hour. Your warm-up would take up the first five to seven minutes. It might begin with a few minutes of some dynamic stretches like swinging your arms in circles, rolling your head on your neck, shaking out and swinging your legs, and other stretches that keep you moving and help you feel loose-limbed and ready for action. Then you might start walking, but slowly, in a leisurely way, maybe combining it with some of those dynamic stretches for the upper body. Then for about twenty minutes you would walk quite briskly at about 80 percent of what you felt was the fastest you could reasonably go, letting yourself feel the momentum and really enjoying moving along at a clip.

As you are getting ready to end, you'd slow down again and then stop walking. Since your muscles would be warm and your blood would be pumping, it'd be a good time to do some more stretching, this time the static kind where you lean into a stretch, stretch as far as you can, and hold it for a few breaths before releasing. You'd probably want to stretch out the backs of your legs especially, since those can get tight when you're walking fast, and do some twists so that your torso and hips would feel nice and loose after walking instead of taut and stiff. The slowing down followed by stretching would let you cool down and let your heart rate come back down to normal, and you'd finish your session feeling like you'd come full circle. How long this takes will vary from person to person and also depends on what kind of activities you've been engaging in, but five to seven minutes of cool-down is a good duration to shoot for.

This warm-up/intense activity/cool-down structure is a classic for a reason, but it is not the only option. Sometimes it is perfectly okay not to warm up separately. You can simply start moving and let your body naturally dictate when and how you intensify your movement as you go. When you want to go out for a walk, you can, but don't have to, spend ten minutes warming up first. You can just put on your walking shoes and head out the door. You might notice that after a few minutes, you pick up your pace and begin to walk faster as your body warms up to the idea. Or you might find that you instinctively choose a moderate pace and just keep going. Both are fine. If your goal is just to move your body and not to achieve a specific fitness goal during that session, there's no reason you have to push in any particular direction. After all, any movement you do will help to at least maintain your physical condition. If you push a little, it will help improve it.

A third potential pattern for structuring a movement session is a warm-up followed by a series of short alternating periods of more, then less, intense movement. This is the format that is used for what is called "interval training," which is often employed when people are trying to achieve rapid progress in particular parameters of their fitness. The popular "One Hundred Push Ups" and "Couch-to-5K" fitness programs both use interval-training methodology to help people ramp up rapidly.

This is simple to apply to a workout of your own devising. You might, following a warm-up, alternate several minutes of moderately brisk walking with several minutes of walking as fast as you possibly can, and cycle back and forth between those things for as long as you wanted your session to continue. Or you might choose a bicycle route featuring a number of short steep hills so you would alternate intense work going up the hills with much less intense work going down the other sides. In the pool, you might alternate stints of leisurely breaststroke and full-out front crawl. There are lots of potential ways to alternate intense and leisurely effort.

You can also combine workout structures if you like. If you've been cruising along at a moderate pace and suddenly feel like going full tilt for a little bit, there's no reason not to. If you've been working pretty hard and feel like a long, slow, tapering cool-down would feel good to you, why not? If you've been doing intervals for a while and feel like switching to a moderate pace and sticking with it for a time, no one is going to stop you, and you cannot possibly do yourself any harm.

Two Sample Workouts

You don't have to have a workout plan in order to move your body. Intuitive movement—just going and doing what feels good—is actually a totally legitimate way to go about getting more movement into your life. You need not target any particular part of your anatomy, tether yourself to a treadmill, or painstakingly distribute your effort among each and every one of your major muscle groups to reap the benefits of increased physical activity. Nevertheless, having an outline of a workout can be useful for reference and as a base on which to build, which can be reassuring and helpful, especially when you're just starting out.

A Baby-Steps Workout

If you're very new to moving your body and starting from a place where you get little physical movement in your day-to-day life, set aside about a half an hour and try the following:

- Stand up and stretch your arms way above your head, reaching for the ceiling. Let yourself droop forward and down until you are stretching toward the floor. Slowly come back up until you are standing up straight, then raise your arms to shoulder level, straight out, and twist your body so that your arms swing around like helicopter blades, back and forth, five times to each side. Come back to the middle, raise your arms again, and repeat the cycle a total of three times.

- Walk at a comfortable pace for five minutes. Just walking around in your house is fine, or go outside and walk down the block for a bit, then work your way back.

- Holding on to the back of a chair, a countertop, or a table, and facing parallel to the chair back, counter, or table, swing your outside leg back and forth without bending your knee. Let the weight of your leg help determine the length of the swing. Don't force it; just let it swing. Do this ten times on each side. Then do the same, but raise your knee as you swing forward, and bend your knee as you swing back. Do this ten times on each side as well. Do another set of each, first with the leg straight, then with the leg bent.
- Walk at a comfortable pace for another five minutes.
- Sit down in a sturdy chair or bench, but do not lean back. Clasp your hands together across your belly and stand back up without using your hands. If this feels unsafe to you, put your hands on some nearby supportive surface (arms of the chair, edge of the chair, etc.) but try not to use them to lever yourself up. Sit back down, controlling your movement so that you don't crash down onto the seat. Sit down and stand up five times.
- Walk at a comfortable pace for another five minutes.
- Finally, sit down on your sturdy chair again. Sit at the edge of the chair, so your sit bones are solidly on the chair. Spread your knees as wide as you comfortably can. Lean forward between your knees, leaning as far as you can comfortably manage, and then come back up so that you are sitting with a straight spine. Breathe in as you come up, and out as you lean forward. Do this five times.

The Ten-Minute Special

This is a workout designed for people who are used to having a more consistent level of moderate activity in their lives. This is for those days when you really don't feel like working out but think you can maybe do it in ten-minute increments because, after all, you can do *anything* for ten minutes.

It is easiest to do this at a gym, but you can do it at home as well if you have some hand weights or something like canned goods or water jugs that you can use as a substitute for hand weights. You will also need a watch or a timer.

- For your first ten minutes, walk at a very deliberate moderate pace. For the first five minutes, swing your arms as much as you can as you walk.

For the second five minutes, consciously lift your knees a bit higher than you usually do as you walk.

- For your second ten minutes, grab your hand weights. Do three sets of ten bicep curls for each arm. Next, still holding those weights, bend forward at the waist and raise your arm out to the side so that it is in a straight line with your shoulder, bring the arm back down, and repeat ten times on each side. Do three sets total. Finally, stand straight up with your feet shoulder-width apart and use the weights to help you stretch first to one side, then the other. Let your shoulder drop, and imagine that the weight is pulling your arm down the side of your leg. Let it pull you as far as you can comfortably go, then come back up slowly to a neutral standing position. Do this five times per side and three sets total.

- For your third ten minutes, choose a higher-intensity aerobic activity: walking briskly, riding a bicycle or exercise bike at a similar speed, or using an elliptical or arc trainer at a reasonably swift pace.

- Your fourth ten minutes are when you bust out your core-strengthening moves. Sit on the edge of a chair, on a bench, or on the floor and hold your hand weights in front of your breastbone, with your elbows bent and out to your side like wings. Lean back slightly and twist your torso to one side, then the other, bringing each elbow as far toward the opposite knee as you can. Do this ten times, give yourself a ten-second break, then do it four more times, giving yourself a ten-second break between sets. After that, if you are comfortable getting down on the floor, get down on your belly and put your arms, elbows bent, by your sides so that your palms are flat on the floor and more or less under your shoulders. Push your torso up as you arch your back up, as if you were trying to touch the ceiling with the top of your forehead. Hold for five seconds, then lower yourself back down; repeat four more times for a set. Do three sets. If you're not comfortable getting down on the floor, clasp your hands behind your back (if this is difficult, grasp both ends of a rolled-up towel or a yoga strap instead) and lean back, thinking about pushing your hands toward the backs of your ankles. Hold for five seconds, then straighten up again. Repeat as above.

- Your fifth ten-minute set will be another moderate- to high-intensity cardio stint of walking (or jogging if you like), biking, elliptical, or the like.

- For your final ten minutes, take the time to stretch out thoroughly. Whatever stretches you like are fine, but make sure to end by letting yourself flop over from the waist, arms dangling down, and give your arms a good shake. Let them hang heavy from your arm sockets. Sometimes your back will make crunchy noises as it realigns itself when you do this. Come up slowly, let your shoulders sink down nice and easy, shake yourself out, give your head a nice leisurely roll around on your shoulders to eliminate neck tension, and you're done!

Modifying Movements

Almost everyone who engages in physical activity engages, whether they know it or not, in a certain amount of movement modification. Left to our own devices, we naturally tend to alter movement to suit our bodies, our strengths, and our preferences. This is why, for example, not everyone walks with the same gait or even picks up a bag of groceries in exactly the same way. Different people and different bodies find their way to subtly different movements, even if they're superficially similar.

The relationship between modifying movements and proper exercise form is a little complex. Proper form is a good idea when we're moving our bodies. It helps us avoid injury and strengthen the parts of our bodies we mean to strengthen. But what if your body won't allow you to do a particular exercise with the canonical version of "proper form"? What do you do if some part of your body simply gets in the way? How do you work with—or around—a big belly, thick thighs, big breasts, wide hips, a big butt?

The answer is that you get creative and you get smart. The goal of a particular exercise—let's say a particular yoga pose—is to involve particular muscles and joints in particular ways. Think about the pose. What parts of the body are moving and where are they supposed to move to? What is meant to be stretching? What is meant to be working harder to hold you up or help you keep your balance?

Now see if you can move your own body to get the same effects. Note that I say *effects* and not *appearance*. Forcing yourself into a position that just *looks* like the ideal version isn't necessarily going to actually produce the right effects anyway, if you're exerting extra force that isn't a part of the original exercise in order to achieve a particular position. If you can't raise your leg all the way to hip level, raise it to knee level. If you can't bend over and touch the floor, bend over and touch your shins, or your knees. If you can't fold your arms in front of your breasts, raise your arms to shoulder-top level and try that. The motions you make should be similar in nature but different in degree. It often helps if you think of it as moving *toward* the ideal form or position, but stopping at the point where you can be comfortable and where the position is sustainable for you rather than trying to force it.

In some cases, there are pieces of equipment that can help you modify movements. Yoga blocks and straps help those who do yoga—and plenty of other kinds of stretching—to achieve positions they can't otherwise manage by offering additional reach and support. Chairs, step aerobics steps, benches, and sturdy wooden boxes of various heights are other useful tools. You can use tightly rolled towels to provide support under your hips or knees or shoulders for floor exercises.

Think outside the box! After I broke my tailbone and discovered I could no longer tolerate doing crunches or sit-ups on a flat surface, even with a yoga mat, I discovered that I could do sit-ups while sitting on a fitness ball just fine. While recovering from a knee injury and temporarily sidelined from several exercises I enjoyed because I couldn't put weight on my knees in an all-fours position, I figured out that I could do reasonably similar exercises draped over a bench. When my belly gets in the way of my doing stretches that are meant to be done with feet together, I just do them with my feet shoulder width apart—which is more stable for me anyway in terms of balance—and stretch into the move as far as I can.

It's *your* body. Don't let a "my way or the highway" attitude about physical form get in the way of your getting the kind of movement you want and need. Pay attention, think carefully about what you're trying to achieve with a particular movement, and then get creative to get your body to do as much of that as possible, within the bounds of your own particular body's abilities. It is totally reasonable, and totally possible, to reenvision form to fit your body.

PLAY TO YOUR STRENGTHS

You wouldn't use an antique Bugatti to tow a trailer full of lawnmowers. You wouldn't try to drive a Grand Prix race in a cement truck. Bodies are not so different. Different people and different bodies have different strengths and weaknesses, and the better you understand your particular body, the better you can play to your strengths.

This is, by the way, entirely okay. Sometimes people feel, for some reason, that they must push themselves ruthlessly to do things that their bodies really aren't all that well suited to doing. Someone who has inherited arthritis and joint problems from both parents, but who feels like the only kind of exercise that counts for anything is training for a marathon, for instance, is probably creating trouble for herself. Someone whose depth perception and hand-eye coordination have never been very good is likely to get frustrated playing squash. This isn't so unlike trying to tow that trailer of lawnmowers with the roadster that was never built for it. It would be a shame for these two hypothetical people to injure and frustrate themselves because they didn't take a step back and appreciate themselves as the very specific makes and models of human being that they are.

As you develop your body practice, take the time to notice what comes easily to your body and what doesn't, what kinds of skills your body acquires quickly and what you struggle with. Figuring out what kind of "vehicle" you have for a body really helps when it comes to figuring out what kinds of activity will help keep it happy and sassy. It doesn't matter one bit what that is. It's totally okay to be a Ferrari, and to have a body that likes going fast—running or rollerblading, for instance—but that might not be terribly good at the hairpin turns of yoga or Pilates. It's equally fine to be a Peterbilt truck and be excellent at lifting heavy things and having the stamina to keep moving all day—which might make you a fantastic hiker or long-distance swimmer—but not to be great at the kinds of bursts of speed and maneuverability that you'd need for, let's say, basketball. And if you're a Honda Civic—not particularly fast and not particularly nimble but you can get the job done—that's actually kind of awesome, because in addition to not being high-maintenance or requiring highly specialized circumstances in order to shine, you're versatile enough to enjoy plenty of variety in your day-to-day exercise life.

It's great to improve your skills and it's great to get stronger and more competent at a range of physical activities. But not all bodies will do all things equally well. Part of developing a good body practice is developing an awareness of what your body does well . . . and learning how to play to those strengths. Why not? It's not like anyone gives you extra purity points for doing things you hate and that make you struggle. There's just no point in punitively forcing yourself to do things you really are not ever going to be constitutionally well suited to doing. Find out what it takes to get you cruising, and you'll be rockin' down the highway for a good long time.

Managing Your Expectations

Moving your body regularly and thoroughly can do a lot of things for you. But it has its limits.

There are limits to what any body practice can do for you, no matter how hard you try, no matter how much effort you put into it, no matter how "virtuous" it seems to be. There will be limits to what your body practice can do for you at any given time in your life. There will be limits to what it can do for you overall.

This is natural, normal, and completely okay. We are, after all, human. Our bodies and our brains are not unlimited resources.

For this very simple reason, we have to be careful of the temptation to believe that we can actually be superhuman if we only go about it the right way. We have to be skeptical of the claims of the fitness-industry ads that promise instant bursts of energy that will turn you into a veritable tornado or that promise magical changes in body shape or size. We need to look very carefully at claims that movement will cure particular diseases, or prevent them. We have to take with an enormous boulder of salt anyone who tries to tell us that our physical activity is a good indicator of our moral uprightness or our general grooviness as human beings. We owe it to ourselves to have a healthy disbelief in the idea that whether and how we move our bodies is going to make other people like us better or think we're better people.

Moving your body is, without question and without qualifications, good for you. Like sleeping, getting enough water to drink and enough food to eat, getting to spend time with people you love, making sure you

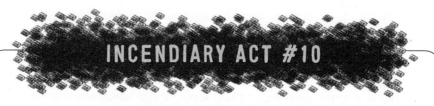

INCENDIARY ACT #10

DARE TO *NOT* COMPARE

Imagine how much easier your life would be if you didn't have to worry about how your performance measured up against everyone else's. How much freer would you feel, knowing that it really didn't matter how what you were doing compared to what other people were doing? Wouldn't it be great if you could judge your own progress based solely on your own past performance, with no one trying to shove some arbitrary external standard down your throat?

When it comes to movement, exercise, and body practice, this is totally achievable.

Keeping your eyes on your own paper, as it were, can be a little tricky. It does mean giving up the easy ego boost of comparing yourself to someone who isn't doing as well as you are. Even harder, it also means giving up the easy bash-yourself-when-you're-feeling-crappy trick, where you deliberately compare yourself to someone who's doing a lot more than you or doing it better.

But in exchange for giving up comparing yourself to other people, you get a wonderful gift: you get to stop comparing yourself to other people. You get to appreciate what you're doing, and how you're doing it, for itself. You get to embrace yourself and your abilities where they are instead of needing to feel superior, or even inferior, to anyone else.

It's remarkably liberating to stop comparing yourself to others. It frees you from an insidious and unhelpful practice and, even better, it frees other people too.

have warm enough clothes when the weather is cold and a place to get out of the sun when it's hot, moving your body is one of those things that just makes your physical body work a whole lot better. Helping your body work the best it can: That's the bottom line of what moving your body will do for you.

What else might moving your body do for you? It's actually hard to say. We know in large outline the kinds of things that physical activity does for people. But no one can predict exactly what physical activity will do for any specific person. Bodies are just too individual, and the range of possible responses is too wide.

The speed with which any physical reaction might happen is another thing that we can't forecast very well. For instance, just because some fitness magazine tells you that you'll instantly feel better and have energy and your life will become an all-singing, all-dancing medley of exuberance the instant you so much as walk around the block doesn't mean it's true. (They mean well. They do. It's supposed to be motivational. But they still lie.) You *may* feel instantly more energetic as soon as you add more activity to your body practice, and if you do, that's fabulous. But it may take a while for the Energy Fairy to show up . . . and even when he does, he may not fork over quite as much of the good stuff as you were hoping. A lot of people find that their energy level increases gradually over time, as the body becomes accustomed to the new situation, rather than changing suddenly. That kind of change may be something you only notice in retrospect.

People's energy levels adjust themselves in the same way that every other parameter of our physical bodies do: as an organic response to changing circumstances and demands. Strength, flexibility, stamina, balance, and everything else about our bodies will adjust themselves as far as they are capable when we make adjustments to our body practice. You can't know in advance how far that will be. But you can let it come as a discovery.

Whether it comes as a pleasant discovery or not is up to you. How you manage your expectations of your body practice makes all the difference. If you can look at the question of "What will the results of this activity be?" with an experimental mind-set rather than with a set of expectations to which you will be holding your body practice hostage, you will very likely feel more successful. It's a matter of looking at things so that you're likely to want what you get, rather than prejudicing the situation so that you will automatically be unhappy if you don't get what you want. With an experimental, discovery-oriented mind-set, you will be able to see the increases in ability and the improvements in the quality of your experience of your own body as positive gains, because they are. You'll be less tempted to generate arbitrary benchmarks for yourself or measure yourself against unrealistic standards that don't really give your poor body much of a chance.

You'll be living in your body for the rest of your life. Treating your body practice and your physical movement as a voyage of discovery rather than a punishing obstacle course is part of the way you can work toward building a real friendship with this thing you'll be spending the rest of your life living with . . . and in. Isn't that a result worth working toward for the long term?

Change Is Inevitable

The only thing that is consistent in life is change. Relationships, jobs, families, our ways of thinking and experiencing the world, and our bodies are all constantly changing, always in at least some minor state of flux. Sometimes the change is slow and steady, other times it is relentless and unpredictable, but there's almost always something somewhere in our lives that is undergoing transition.

Change is also a bit like a line of dominoes: tip one over, and the next gets knocked down, and the next, in turn. When one aspect of our lives changes, others change in response, sometimes harmoniously and sometimes less so.

This is palpably true when it comes to our bodies and movement. Making changes in your body practice and your day-to-day physical life can be wonderful and liberating but also complicated . . . and sometimes unsettling.

It bears remembering that change isn't just the stuff that happens to you or the situations you end up in. It's also things you do yourself, with full intent. Moving your body more, adding motion and physical exertion to your life, constitutes a change. And for every fat girl who leaps into newfound movement with a sense of joy and liberation at finally feeling like she's allowed to do something she's wanted to do for years, there will be those who find the whole issue of adding physical activity to their daily lives so unsettling that they'll have to approach it several times from different angles, stopping and starting and running into walls, before they finally figure out a way to do it so that it doesn't feel too weird to be tolerated.

It is rare that mainstream fitness sources acknowledge that the ways people react to changes in their body practice can be complicated and emotionally difficult. There's a real bias, in the fitness industry, toward thinking about increased movement as an unmitigated good. Actual human beings and their responses are a bit more complicated than this. Actual human beings who also have to grapple with movement histories and memories and experiences that have been made additionally complex by all the social and physical and personal issues that fatness can add can be a *lot* more complicated. Emotional reactions to making a change and adding more movement to your life are natural and normal and understandable. They are legitimate, and it is entirely reasonable that people experience them.

But in the end, a complicated reaction is only a complicated reaction. There's no reason a complicated reaction needs to stop you from doing the things you want to do with your body practice, even if it does give you a lot to think about. It can actually help to move your body while you think through the various reactions you have to doing it; just let the thoughts and feelings bubble up while you move and see what your brain has to say about what your body is doing.

Change is not always immediate. It does not always follow a predictable schedule. It's also not very controllable. Sometimes we wish we could change things about ourselves, or about our reactions, yet we find that we can't change them just because we want to. We can only do the things we need to do and give ourselves some time to adjust. Our attitudes toward changing our body practices are often in that category. Many fat women have endured such trauma around movement and physical activity that the only thing that eventually recalibrates their reactions to even the prospect of movement is a good long while of gently, regularly, engaging in movement without judgment or expectations until it just becomes normal.

Change also comes on multiple fronts when it comes to body practice. There are changes in our emotions and our thoughts. There are changes in our subjective experiences of our bodies. There are also changes in our bodies themselves. Increasing movement will change your body in various ways that can include everything from increases in strength and stability to changes in body shape and proportions to changes in biochemistry and how your body responds to environmental factors like stress or pollution.

We get to choose our voluntary actions. But we do not get to choose every change that happens in our lives, not even where our own personal physical bodies are concerned. Some of the changes we experience, yes, have a certain amount of cause and effect about them: if we do a lot of bicep curls, we are likely to find that our arms get stronger. But we do not necessarily get to choose whether we ever develop sharply defined biceps. Some bodies will, other bodies won't, and still other bodies will only do so under very specific additional conditions. Our bodies, ultimately, decide what they will do or not do with the raw materials we give them, and that very much includes the physical activity we engage in.

Chosen or not, and even visible or not, the changes that come along with increasing your movement and your physical activity can be tricky to negotiate, emotionally and socially. Give yourself a chance to experience the changes that come your way, to think about them and see if there aren't positive things to be had from the experience. Sure, sometimes you'll freak out, but that's not the end of the world. Eventually, you'll stop freaking out . . . and that way, perspective lies.

What's Buzzin' Cousin?

What's buzzing around inside you as you move? Especially if moving your body regularly is a new thing for you, it might be hard to parse what's going on in your head when you do it. The following is a little series of questions that might help you zero in on some of it:

- What word pops into your head when you think about what it feels like to get ready to go move and be physically active?

- What three physical sensations do you most strongly associate with starting to move your body during any given stint of movement?

- What three physical sensations do you most strongly associate with being in the middle of a period of physical activity?

- Does engaging in physical activity, at this point in your life, bring up any memories for you? If so, of what or whom? Does it differ depending on what activity you're doing?

- What do you want to say to someone when you're moving your body? What sorts of things do you imagine being able to tell people?

- What one word pops into your head when you are just finished with a session of physical movement?

Pay attention to these answers. They might tell you that you are, for instance, feeling some fear as you start, but that it gets easier. They might tell you that you're experiencing some sensations of helplessness that get replaced by anger or rebellion. They might inform you that every time you get on the treadmill, you think about that sleazy diet doctor your mom took you to when you were fourteen, but that when you use the rowing machine, you feel like a world-conquering gladiator. They may present you with the pleasant surprise that you're finding something freeing and delightful about movement, but that it's still a little scary, and so on. The things that come up for you are bound to change over time. Checking in with these kinds of questions on a regular basis is a great way to keep your fingers on the pulse of your own relationship to your body practice as you grow, change, and get stronger.

Wanted Versus Unwanted Changes

One of the few things you can count on in this life is that most people enjoy getting what they want and don't like getting what they don't want. When it comes to the changes created by increasing your physical activity, we can end up feeling simultaneously rewarded and challenged, and at other times punished, by the kinds of things that change and how other people react to those changes.

Wanted Changes Are the Simplest Ones to Negotiate

If you want to increase your strength and flexibility and then you work at it and your body changes to become stronger and more flexible, then you got what you wanted. Good on you!

But even such wanted changes can get complicated when other people start chiming in. What you want for yourself and what other people want for you don't always match up. Someone warning you not to do too much strength training—"You don't want to bulk up!"—just when you're starting to feel good about your increased strength is really not helping matters. When people feel that noticing a change in your body entitles them to an opinion, it can really make things uncomfortable.

Having to learn how to disengage when other people feel the need to impose their thoughts and priorities on you does not exactly reduce your stress levels. But realistically speaking, you are going to end up having to negotiate other people's reactions to your body no matter what you do. (Surely you have noticed that even if your body doesn't change, people sometimes feel the need to share unsolicited opinions about it.) So you may as well do the things you want to do with your body regardless. At least that way you get to do what you want, and what helps you achieve your own priorities as far as what you want your body to be able to be and do.

Unwanted Changes Are Tougher by Far

Unwanted changes are tougher because there's friction on all sides of the equation. Sometimes our bodies do things we'd really rather they not, and when they do, it hardly matters why. It can feel like you've been betrayed by your own body. This is not the same as feeling like you've let yourself down or disappointed yourself, because an unwanted bodily change is hardly something you did intentionally. Our bodies have minds of their own sometimes, and that's exactly what's so hard to cope with.

So what do you do if, let's say, your new body practice leaves you with pants that no longer fit because your thighs have actually gotten bigger because they've become substantially more muscular? What do you do if you discover, as some people do, that with increased movement, your body informs you in no uncertain terms that you have a temperamental joint that

FOCUS ON WHAT MAKES YOU FIERCE

The only thing that really counts, as far as the results of your body practice are concerned, is whether or not you feel fierce. If what you do makes you feel great, if it makes you stronger and more capable of dealing with your life and your body and being in the world, if it makes you feel like you're brighter and shinier and ready to stir things up, *that's what matters.*

You're the only person who has to live in your body. You're the only person who gets to decide what makes you feel fierce and what doesn't. Other people can have all the opinions they want. You're still the only person whose vote actually counts. Focusing on what makes you feel fierce, what makes you feel fantastic and fine and full of beans, is the single best way to gauge whether or not you're doing what's right for your body.

There are a lot of different ways you can move your body, get stronger, improve your stamina, work on your balance, become more flexible, and all the rest of it. Every time you turn around, it seems, someone is trying to tell you that one particular sport or type of exercise machine or fitness class or athletic endeavor is the be-all and end-all. That's fine, and it's great if it works that way for them. But if you try it out and it really doesn't do it for you—oh well! People are different. Just because it works for one person doesn't mean it'll work for everybody. If yoga classes don't make you feel fierce, that's okay. Maybe aikido will. Or taking tango classes. Or sea kayaking. Or . . .

The same goes for all the other aspects of your body practice. So what if you read some magazine article somewhere that said that the best time to exercise was between 8 and 10 a.m.? If you try it and all it does for you is make you too zoned out on endorphins to be functional until after lunch, maybe it's not the best time *for you* to exercise. Maybe someone told you that the most effective leg exercise was lunges, but you hate them, they hurt your knees, and they remind you repulsively of high school gym class. Oh well! Fortunately, there are hundreds of ways to exercise your legs. You'll just have to figure out what the best leg exercise in the world is *for you*. Which one is that? Easy: the one that makes your legs feel like *kicking some ass.*

simply has to be babied? How, indeed, do you respond when your body simply fails to change in the ways you'd like and leaves you with the distinct feeling that you've been awfully diligent about your body practice and couldn't your stupid body just cooperate for a change?

And what if, on top of this, other people felt entitled, as they so often do, to chime in? What if they "tsk tsk" about your thick thighs and imply that if you were doing the *correct* exercises, you wouldn't have bulked up like that? What if someone just *has* to go there and tells you that your joint wouldn't be so prone to injury if only you weren't so darned fat? And for heaven's sake, how do you reply to someone who notes that you've been at the gym religiously but you don't look any different, with all the enormous payload of suspicion and disapproval that can be packed into such a statement?

First things first: you go right back to your first principles, your fundamental motivations for moving your body, like strength, stamina, power, peace of mind, a healthier immune system, stress relief, and so on. You can check in with these and see how you've become stronger and more sturdy, the ways in which you feel more serene and powerful.

Then you acknowledge that your body really does have a mind of its own, and your powerful, healthy, strong thighs are going to do whatever they damn well please . . . and you can't actually stop them, and neither can anyone else, so you may as well figure out how to enjoy them. You acknowledge that bodies have needs, and strengthening the muscles and tendons that support those sometimes-cranky joints can only be a good thing that will help make them tougher and more resilient. And what about the people who insinuate that you must somehow be screwing up if you're frequently at the gym but your body hasn't changed in the way they apparently expected it would? Well, the temptation to smile sweetly and say "Yeah, well, you can't necessarily *see* that someone's gotten a whole lot better equipped to kick your ass" is strong, isn't it?

Remember, also, to thank your body for doing all the things it's doing right. It's ungrateful, and really unkind to yourself, to refuse to give yourself credit where credit is due. Your body is doing right by you in every way it knows how. Appreciate the things it does right and the ways that it supports you and improves your life. That's the important stuff, and the rest is largely not anything you can control anyway.

Body Weight and Size Changes

Weight and size changes are among the most difficult and emotionally fraught changes we face in our body practice. The reason rarely has much to do with the actual weight or size. No, the reason weight and size changes are so difficult is that it is all but impossible to think about them in any kind of neutral way. The culture we live in and its relentless focus on body size, shape, and weight pretty much guarantees that neither we nor anyone else is likely to experience a change in weight or size without a strong emotional reaction.

This is a big problem. It means that there is no way to engage in any body practice that might potentially have some effect on your body's shape, size, or appearance without assuming the risk of walking into a hornet's nest of strong, even extreme, responses to your body. This is insidious: it makes it very difficult to form your own independent opinions and have your own authoritative emotions about your body without them having already been tossed around in the storm of other people's perceptions. It's enough, sometimes, to keep people from pursuing a body practice that gives them pleasure and contributes manifestly to their well-being just because it is so damn difficult and painful to run the gauntlet of emotional reactions to potential changes in body shape, size, and appearance.

The elephant in the body-practice room when we talk about increasing physical activity is, of course, weight loss, or, as I prefer to call it, shrinking.

Feelings about the prospect that one's increased physical activity may lead to a change in the weight, size, or shape of one's body run a wide and deeply felt gamut. Some of us are very invested in shrinking and desire it earnestly and powerfully. Others have decided that focusing on it is too painful or presents too much temptation to behave in ways that they know from long experience cause them harm. Some people try not to think about it one way or the other. Still others of us rebel against the notion that every fat person must necessarily want to become thinner, and we actively resist shrinking. Some of us are more laissez-faire. This is actually not an unreasonable stance to take. Bodies are very good at finding their own comfortable resting points. As Kelly Bliss puts it on her blog (Life with Bliss), "take care of your body and let your body take care of your weight." There is room in the world for all these viewpoints. There is also room for viewpoints to change over time.

It seems important in this book, therefore, that we make room for all those viewpoints and more, and that we not dictate how anyone should feel about it if their body should shrink—or enlarge, for that matter—in response to a change in body practice. But it also seems important to acknowledge that we will, almost inevitably, have some feelings about such changes.

It's important to recognize that change always includes loss. Losing a body shape or size with which you were familiar, even if it was not one you particularly liked or even accepted, is still a form of loss. It can feel very strange to look in the mirror or see a picture of yourself and not quite recognize yourself—quite a sensation of whiplash. This can be all the stronger when other people react to your change in body size. This is true both for desired and undesired changes. Any change in your body shape or size can be a double-edged knife. This is especially true for shrinking. Even if you wanted to shrink, having other people congratulate you on doing so can sometimes leave you feeling itchy and weird.

It takes time to adjust to physical change. As we become stronger and fitter, we have to learn how to recalibrate what we do in our physical activity so that it reflects new ability levels. The 80 percent rule (see page 138) is a nice, flexible, even intuitive way to do this, but it still requires that we make adjustments and changes. Changes in the dimensions of our bodies also take time to adjust to . . . and there's no 80 percent rule to help you with that.

People often assume that if your body is changing in a way that is considered desirable, then the change itself will be a source of pleasure. This isn't necessarily true. Having your body be a different size or shape, having it fit into clothes and exercise machines and your car and the pews at church differently than it used to, can feel alienating and stressful until you get used to the new normal. Regardless of the direction of the discrepancy between your self-image and your actual body, it can be uncomfortable when self-image and body do not agree.

Your body will, inevitably, change in shape and size, contour and proportion over the course of your life. It may be linked to your body practice or it may simply be part of the array of Silly Body Tricks that we each experience over time as we age and our bodies change. Letting yourself react to the changes, and simultaneously trying to maintain some sort of sense of separation between your reactions and the reactions of others, are not simple tasks. Shrink or expand, though, it is always your own experience of your body that matters most, no matter how you change.

CHAPTER 6

Troubleshooting

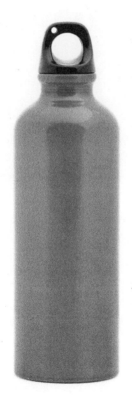

A successful body practice requires that you be your own best advocate, both for your body and your mental health. This section helps you know what you need to know so that you can look out for yourself in a number of crucial ways. From nutrition to warning signs of impending health crisis, sports injuries to fat-bashing, including dealing with doctors in regard to your fitness and your health, having good information at your disposal helps make you a more effective advocate and a more formidable force for fierce fat fitness.

Stop Right There

We experience a wide range of physical sensations and responses when we move our bodies. Some of them are pleasurable, some of them are uncomfortable, and some of them are just odd. Some are transient; others last a while. Most of them you can just note in passing and keep on doing what you're doing.

There are some, however, that should stop you in your tracks. If you experience any of the following sensations or symptoms when you are physically active—or at any time—you should stop what you're doing immediately and seek medical attention. They may be nothing. But they may also be signs of severe potential health crisis, or the existence of a major health crisis in progress:

- Sudden intense pain in the chest, neck, shoulder, or jaw

- Intense pain that radiates out from your chest, either into your arm or up your neck

- Racing heartbeat that does not slow to normal after you stop moving
- Difficulty breathing or difficulty catching your breath again after you stop moving
- Dizziness or vertigo
- Sudden-onset severe headache, visual disturbances, or loss of balance

If you experience any of these, stop what you're doing immediately and seek medical help. Some of these symptoms may indicate heart attack or stroke, and in both cases, time is of the essence. It is always better to be safe than sorry.

Common Sports Injuries and What to Do About Them

There are a range of very common injuries that can happen as a result of physical activity. Most of them are quite minor, but if you aren't familiar with them, even a minor ouch or ailment can seem more serious than it necessarily is. In most cases, it's not only possible but absolutely fine to treat these kinds of minor problems at home by yourself. Knowing some strategies for avoiding them in the first place is even better.

Skin Injuries and Problems

Skin issues include all kinds of scrapes, abrasions, irritations, chafing, blisters, and other unpleasant things. These annoyances are usually fairly minor and heal on their own if you keep them clean and protected, but occasionally they need professional treatment.

Blisters

- **What they are:** A blister is a collection of clear or light yellow fluid under the top layers of skin, which forms a bubble to cushion and protect the underlying tissue against friction, extreme temperature, or other harmful things. Blisters related to physical activity often happen on the feet and toes and sometimes on the hands and fingers.

- **How to treat them:** If the blister is intact, try to leave it that way. Unbroken blisters are protective, and the fluid will reabsorb on its own in a few days if you let it. Simply cover the blister with a bandage and let it heal. If the blister has broken, treat it as you would a cut. Clean the wound, apply some antibiotic ointment, and cover it with a bandage.

- **When to see a doctor:** If the fluid in a blister is clear or yellowish, don't worry about it. Occasionally, you will see a blister filled with blood or bloody fluid. This is also nothing to worry about. However, if the blister appears to be filled with opaque or greenish pus, it may be infected, and you should see a doctor to have it checked out.

- **How to prevent them:** Preventing the friction that causes blisters to form is the key to preventing blisters. Socks that wick away sweat and that fit properly, shoes that fit and are secured properly to the foot, and paying attention to whether or not you are getting "hot spots" of friction when you move are all part of prevention. Sometimes you may want to wear an adhesive bandage or a bit of tape or moleskin to protect vulnerable bits of skin from friction. To avoid blisters on the hands, wear gloves when doing things that are likely to cause a lot of friction such as rowing, raking leaves, and so on.

Chafing

- **What it is:** Chafing, also known among unapologetic fat girls as "chub rub," is the result of friction against the skin that creates a mild abrasion. Skin gets red, tender, and sometimes raw. Lymph scabbing may occur. It is most common on the inner thighs, in the groin, under the arms, and on nipples. Wet skin is more prone to chafing.

- **How to treat it:** Wash the chafed area with mild soap and warm water and pat thoroughly dry. Cover with a thin layer of a neutral but protective ointment such as petroleum jelly, triple antibiotic ointment (or Neosporin), or A & D ointment. Avoid ointments with perfumes and other additives, as they can irritate. Cover the area with a bandage or some gauze. Chafing should heal in a few days, depending on severity.

- **When to see a doctor:** If a chafed area feels very hot and hard to the touch, if it swells, oozes pus, smells bad, is exceptionally painful, or otherwise appears as if it might be infected, see a doctor.

- **How to prevent it:** Wear clothes that fit properly and be attentive to places where clothes bunch or rub you. Keep hydrated so that you will sweat freely. Having sweat dry on your skin can actually increase chafing due to the tiny salt crystals left over from dried sweat, which can irritate. If you have problems with chafing in specific areas, like the infamous inner-thigh zone, there are lubricants like Bodyglide and Sportslick that are made specifically to reduce chafing in high-friction areas. You can buy these at sporting goods or running shops or online. For nipple chafing, try an adhesive bandage or sports tape over the nipples. (Yes, really—it works!)

Muscle and Soft-Tissue Concerns

These injuries and issues range from the superficial to the severe. Soreness, strains, sprains, and other soft-tissue problems should be treated with care and allowed adequate healing time; weak, still-healing muscles and connective tissue are more easily injured than strong, fully healed ones.

Muscle Soreness

- **What it is:** Delayed onset muscle soreness, also called DOMS, is the "morning after" pain you feel in your muscles that sets in following a stint of physical activity. It's caused by a combination of factors, including microscopic tears in the muscles you've used (this is normal and part of how muscles get stronger) and inflammation. It generally goes away on its own if you rest the muscles and let them recover.

- **How to treat it:** Gentle stretching, over-the-counter anti-inflammatories like aspirin or ibuprofen, drinking plenty of water, hot baths/showers, hot compresses or heating pads, and rest. Light exercise that helps keep the muscle moving gently and slowly can help too.

- **When to see a doctor:** If soreness is extreme, lasts more than a few days without improvement, or is accompanied by swelling or the inability to bend or bear weight on an affected body part, see a doctor.

- **How to prevent it:** Dynamic stretching before vigorous physical activity and static stretching during or afterward can help prevent muscle soreness. Having a cool-down phase in your workout also helps muscles return to a resting state more gracefully, which seems to help reduce soreness later.

Shin Splints

- **What they are:** Pain along the shinbone (tibia) of the lower leg, sometimes accompanied by mild swelling, is caused by stress and damage to connective tissues between the bone and the muscles of the lower leg. Sometimes they are caused by specific types of running (or less often, walking), such as running downhill or playing tennis or other sports with a lot of fast stops, starts, and turns. Poor shoes with inadequate support can also contribute to shin splints, particularly if you have flat feet or are engaging in a lot of high-impact activities.

- **How to treat them:** Rest! Avoid doing the things that cause you shin splints. If you still want to move your body, swimming and biking are good options, and activities like yoga may also feel good and not aggravate the inflammation. Ice the affected area for up to twenty minutes at a time to reduce swelling and take an over-the-counter painkiller like aspirin or ibuprofen. Wear good supportive shoes to help keep from reinjuring the shin while it heals.

- **When to see a doctor:** If there is a great deal of swelling or things do not begin to improve in a week or so, see a doctor. Occasionally, a stress fracture can masquerade as shin splints.

- **How to prevent them:** Wear proper, well-fitting shoes with good support. Arch supports can help distribute stress better across your entire foot, which means that the shin has less to absorb. Choose low- or moderate-impact activities and avoid running or walking too hard, too fast, or too far for comfort.

Plantar fasciitis

- **What it is:** Plantar fasciitis is intense heel pain caused by the inflammation of a band of tissue, the plantar fascia, that wraps around the bottom of the foot from the base of the toes to the back of the heel. People experiencing plantar fasciitis often report that the first few steps in the morning (or after a long period of sitting) are excruciating, but that after the foot has had a chance to acclimatize to bearing weight, it is not as bad. Interestingly, plantar fasciitis tends to affect only one foot at a time. Women are more likely to get it than men.

- **How to treat it:** Over-the-counter painkillers (aspirin, ibuprofen) are useful. You can also ice the bottom of the foot. Some people have success using a frozen bottle of water as a hard roller against which to press the foot, rolling the foot back and forth to simultaneously ice and stretch the plantar fascia. Make sure that your shoes are supportive and fit properly and that they have good arch support. Switch to lower-impact activities. Put your feet up and let the swelling and inflammation have a chance to recede for a while.

- **When to see a doctor:** If you are unable to generate improvement even with good and properly supporting shoes, regular stretching, icing, and a switch to low- or nonimpact movement, see a doctor.

- **How to prevent it:** Properly supportive shoes with good arch support are crucial. Going barefoot, for some people, may be a trigger for plantar fasciitis. Stretching the fascia on a regular basis, for instance, by standing with your toes on the edge of a step and then letting your heels sink down below the level of your toes, can help, as can flexing the toes up toward the shin by other methods. A doctor may recommend a night splint to stretch the fascia while you sleep or that orthotics be inserted into shoes for improved support during the day.

Strains and Sprains

- **What they are:** Strains are the overstretching or tearing of muscles or tendons. (Tendons are the connective tissues that connect muscles to bones.) Symptoms of strains include pain, swelling, bruising, and a limited ability to use the affected joint. You may also experience muscle spasms.

  Sprains are the overstretching or tearing of ligaments, the tough bands of connective tissue that are in your joints, connecting one bone to the next. Symptoms of sprains include pain, swelling, bruising, and limited or no ability to use the affected joint. You may hear a "pop" noise at the time of injury.

- **How to treat them:** Sprains and strains are treated best with the RICE protocol: **r**est, **i**ce, **c**ompression (elastic bandage or ACE bandage wrap), and **e**levation. Additionally, take over-the-counter painkillers as required. Strains and sprains usually heal in three to six weeks. You may want to wear a brace during the latter part of the healing period for a sprain to provide additional support until you get to the point where you feel the body part has become strong enough to trust it fully again.

- **When to see a doctor:** Mild strains and sprains can be treated at home. But if you can't move the affected body part at all, cannot put weight on it, or have numbness in the affected area, see a doctor. Also see a doctor if the pain is exceptionally severe or if it becomes worse over time instead of better.

- **How to prevent them:** Build strength slowly and consistently rather than pushing yourself too far at any one time. Stronger muscles, tendons, and connective tissues are less likely to get injured than weak ones. Be sure to warm up properly before you try vigorous activity and be careful of sudden stops, starts, turns, and twists.

Skeletal Concerns

Bones are sturdy but not invulnerable, and bone-related injuries need special care to heal properly. Do not hesitate to seek medical attention for these issues.

Stress Fractures

- **What they are:** Stress fractures are tiny cracks in a bone caused by repetitive stress or overuse, such as hard pounding of the feet during running or jumping. They're most common in the legs and feet. They have many of the same symptoms as strains and sprains, including pain, swelling, tenderness, and so on, but are not limited to joint areas. Because incompletely healed stress fractures tend to get worse with further exercise of the type that caused them in the first place, the pain often increases over time.

- **How to treat them:** You can use over-the-counter painkillers (or prescription if a doctor indicates), the RICE protocol outlined above, and whatever physical therapy or assistive devices a doctor may prescribe, such as crutches, a walking boot, or a brace.

- **When to see a doctor:** Stress fractures can be deceptively tricky and easily mistaken for sprains and strains. The red flag to watch for is pain that does not go away with substantial rest.

- **How to prevent them:** Pay attention to the pain. If pain is getting more severe as you continue to work out over time, you may have a problem on your hands. Otherwise, proper footwear, good nutrition for strong bones, strength training for more muscular support, and a gentle approach to being active without overdoing it are your best bets.

SOME INSIDER SECRETS FOR HAPPIER BODY PRACTICE FROM THE ANCIENT AND EXALTED SISTERHOOD OF INCENDIARY FAT-GIRL EXERCISERS

1. If you are prone to minor muscle or joint pain while you move your body, take a normal dose of an over-the-counter anti-inflammatory painkiller like aspirin or ibuprofen half an hour before you plan to exercise to help smooth your progress.

2. Can't get your rings off after a workout? If you find your fingers swell when you're exercising, it is likely because you're not moving your arms enough to keep blood from pooling in your hands and lower forearms. Get your arms up above your shoulders and wiggle them around, or do jumping jacks or windmill-style arm movements while you're doing other things, particularly if you're doing leg-based cardio like walking or biking.

continued

---

3. Don't let an elliptical trainer, stair climber, or exercise bike carry you off into a too-fast whizzing oblivion just because your weight on the pedals makes them move more quickly than you expected. The culprit is usually a too-low resistance level. Increasing the machine's resistance level so that it is a better match for the weight you are bringing to bear on the situation will allow you to choose a speed that better suits your abilities without being rushed by gravity.

4. Adjust your shoes as you proceed during a workout. Feet sweat, and may sometimes also swell, during movement. If your feet are bothering you, or it begins to feel like your athletic shoes don't fit, take a moment to completely remove, then put on, your shoes, adjusting the laces or straps so that your shoes are comfortable but still supportive.

5. Exercising in the evening often has a paradoxical effect: you think it'll tire you out, but instead you end up with a second wind that ruins your sleep schedule and leaves you dragging the next day. Even nonvigorous exercise, like tai chi or yoga, can do this. If you're prone to such bursts of postmovement energy, it helps to make sure you finish your workout at least three hours before you need to be in bed, giving the uncontrollable jazz hands some time to run their course.

6. If you are prone to swollen legs or feet, or to varicose veins, end your movement session with ten minutes of lying down with your feet higher than your head. Prop them up against a bench, chair, wall, Swiss ball, or whatever is convenient. (This is a great time to do some arm exercises with hand weights, by the way.) Swimming is also fantastic for anyone prone to any form of swelling or edema in the extremities. Water pressure creates fantastic gentle compression and supports lymph and blood circulation.

7. Dusting powder (cornstarch or talc) works great for preventing chub rub . . . but only if you don't get too sweaty. Heavy sweating plus powder plus friction creates something that looks and feels a lot like modeling clay and

collects in skin creases, where it doesn't do a damn thing to prevent skin friction. A better bet, if you're going to be sweating a lot, are lubricants like Bodyglide. Shower after you're done, dry off completely, then use powder.

8. Got crotch rot? Minor fungal infections in skin folds are pretty common among athletes of all sizes, but especially those of us with more skin folds than the average person. If things in your armpits or below the belt are a little itchy and a little yeasty-smelling, you may be able to avoid a doctor's office trip by washing carefully, drying completely, then treating the affected parts several times a day with over-the-counter creams sold for treating vaginal yeast infections. Do see a doctor if it doesn't clear up in a few days, though, as it may not be a bug that the cream in question is capable of treating.

9. Women are often more prone to musculoskeletal injury when they are menstruating or about to menstruate, due to hormone fluctuations that can loosen connective tissues. Be extra careful of your joints when Flo Crampton and her Red River Blues Band are playing at a venue near you. If you have joints that have a history of significant weakness or major injury, consider using light-duty supportive braces or athletic tape to support them during that time of your cycle.

10. Skirts are superbly comfortable exercise wear. They don't bind or limit your motion, don't ride up between your legs like some pairs of shorts can, don't bunch at the groin, and you can't beat the air circulation. They can also be a godsend if you are freaked out about having people see too much of your butt, belly, hips, or thighs. Wear bike shorts underneath to avoid chub rub, or liberally deploy the antifriction balm of your choice to whatever parts of you require it.

Getting What You Came for at the Doctor's

When you are fat, it can be hard to get what you came for at the doctor's office. Instead of treating whatever it was that brought you into their office, many doctors want to focus on your weight. (Telling you you're fat is, after all, the easiest medical diagnosis in the world. All the doctor has to do is look at you.) So how can you best ensure that you get what you came for when you go to the doctor?

Know Why You're Going

Do your homework and be able to state what you want clearly. Direct statements and clear requests are better than passive descriptions and vague hand waving. For example, say,

> *"I twisted my right ankle in aerobics class yesterday. It may be sprained. I can put some weight on it, but it is very painful. The outside edge of the ankle is swollen worse than the inside"*

and not

> *"Well, my ankle really hurts. I guess I did something to it. I don't know. It happened in aerobics class and it hurts a lot."*

The former gives your doctor information and makes you part of a collaborative process. It tells your doctor what happened, what part of the body was affected, how long ago the injury happened, how you injured it, what your symptoms are like, what you've observed about the injury, and your sense of what kind of injury it might be. The second approach does not give much information; it just tells your doctor you've got some pain and swelling in your ankle and that whatever happened, happened in aerobics class. The former approach tells your doctor that you have put some thought into what's going on, have an informed opinion, and can be trusted as a reliable witness of your own physical condition. The latter just communicates that you're in pain and you want the doctor to make it better.

Know What You Want

Again, this requires some forethought. Do you want a diagnosis? Do you just want it to stop hurting? Do you need help figuring out how to avoid making it worse or reinjuring yourself? You might be looking for some sort of assistive device or a referral to a specialist or physical therapist. Practice asking focused questions, like these:

- "Does this seem like a strain to you or a sprain?"
- "Will I need to wear this brace at night or only during the daytime?"
- "How will I know when it's okay to use this arm normally again?"
- "I'm having a lot of trouble sleeping because of the pain; what can I do about that?"
- "I'm afraid of making this worse. What should I be doing to make sure I don't?"
- "Could you recommend a specialist I could talk to about this?"

Be Prepared to Redirect the Conversation

If your practitioner veers away from the reason you've established for your visit, feel free to direct him or her right back. Reminding the practitioner why you are in the examining room is totally appropriate. Active listening techniques can be helpful: acknowledge that the practitioner has mentioned something else, then steer the conversation back where it belongs. For example, you can say, "Yes, that is correct: I am fat. That is not my medical concern today, though. My medical concern today is my dislocated thumb."

More than one redirection may be required. Sometimes it is useful to point out that your weight, whatever your doctor may think of it, is a separate issue and not one that is going to change in the time it takes to diagnose and treat what brought you into the office. "Yes, I am fat, but I am not going to become slim right this minute. Right this minute, I need you to treat my dislocated thumb." Remind them, firmly and repeatedly if necessary, of what you need: a diagnosis, a medication, a treatment, a referral, and so on.

Be Prepared to Challenge Blaming Behaviors

A practitioner may chide you for an injury and claim that you would not have injured yourself if you were not fat. Blaming someone for her own injury or illness is not helpful or productive. You are totally within your rights to point out that slender people also get injured when they are engaging in physical activity. It happens all the time. Your injury is actually no different. The only thing that is different is that you are being blamed for it, and that is unfair.

You are also totally within your rights to point out that given the choice between a fat patient who exercises, and thus takes the risk that she might get injured in the process, and a fat patient who never exercises and thus never runs the risk of any related injury, most doctors would prefer the former. No doctor should be blaming you for an injury, but if one does, it's fair play to dish it right back.

Additionally, you should know that *you do not have to consent to be weighed*. Many people find it traumatic (the result of many years of bad experiences) to be asked to step on a scale in a doctor's office. It is okay to say, "I prefer not to be weighed." It is also acceptable to tell your doctor that should he or she need to weigh you for the purposes of prescribing a weight-based dosage or something else where a weight number is immediately relevant, you will be happy to cooperate, but that if all they're doing is collecting statistics, you'd rather not subject yourself to the psychological trauma of being weighed. I have been known to say I have PTSD—which I explain stands for "post-traumatic scale disorder"—half-jokingly getting the point across.

Strategic Advisors

If you are coping with a chronic health condition, injury, or disability, you may need to consult with a strategic advisor about what kinds of movement will work best for you and how you can best perform them so that you support and improve your health rather than undermine it. Normal athletic coaches and standard-issue personal trainers may not be qualified to work with special medical needs. You may need to consult a specialist to help you brainstorm, invent, and strategize ways to move your body safely and happily. The following are some of the types of specialists you might consider:

- **Sports medicine physicians.** These are doctors who may be general practitioners or in another specialty (commonly orthopedics) who have an additional subspecialty in sports medicine and the treatment of athletes and their particular injuries and issues. They diagnose and treat a wide range of sports-related injuries and problems, often with the aid of one or more types of the practitioners listed below.

- **Physical therapists.** These are medical professionals who work with doctors and other health care practitioners, but who are also qualified to diagnose and treat a range of issues affecting body posture, alignment, mobility, and physical well-being using a variety of nonsurgical and nonpharmaceutical methods. Their focus, in general, is on functional fitness—the ability to carry out normal life activities successfully. There are physical therapists who specialize in sports medicine as well.

- **Rehabilitative or medical exercise specialists.** These are personal trainers whose primary training is in fitness, but who have additional medicalized training that lets them work with clients as an adjunct to medical treatment. They assist people who have already begun the process of healing from an illness, injury, or treatment (such as cardiac surgery or cancer treatment) to strengthen and rebuild bodies that have been challenged in particular medical ways. They function in a rehabilitative role, working to get clients as strong and as fit as possible given their particular medical histories. They are also trained to watch for warning signs that a client may need additional medical treatment or care. They differ from physical therapists in that their training is not fundamentally medical in nature, and they cannot diagnose or treat illness or injury, only help to strengthen and support healing that is already being overseen by medical professionals.

Nutrition and the Active Eater

It seems like virtually everyone from your coworkers to your doctor to your mom is certain, in their heart of hearts, that they are among the world's leading authorities on nutrition. This isn't a big surprise. Fueled by innumerable breathless headlines about studies that have determined that if you eat nine pounds of broccoli a day, you will never get sick; that vitamin D is the secret to eternal life; or that women need to constantly consume dairy products or their bones will crumble to dust as soon as menopause hits, *et very much cetera*, most of us acquire a collection of beliefs about the secret rules of "eating right."

And eating right, we often believe, is all-important. However we might define "eating right" for the moment, we tend to believe that it is the key to perfect health, perfect bodies, and a form of moral virtue as well. It's not. But it's also not too surprising that we tend to get just the tiniest bit overinvested in largely notional food rules.

You don't need to do this to yourself. Honest, you really don't. Most food "rules" can simply, and safely, be ignored. They're not usually very sound from a biological perspective, and though few of them are likely to hurt you seriously, they're also not particularly likely to help.

Fortunately, eating well and nourishing your body properly for an active and engaged life is easier for most people to do than you might think. There are just a few very basic principles to follow.

Make Sure You're Getting Enough to Eat

We need enough food to function properly. We need food for energy—it's what keeps us warm, keeps our brains working, and lets us move around—but we also need food to keep our muscles and bones and brains and internal organs well supplied with all the things they need so they can do what they're supposed to do. When we don't get enough to eat, we may still be able to function, but we probably won't be functioning as well as we could. This is no good! The world is a challenging place, and to thrive in it, we need to function at our best as much of the time as we can. Give yourself a chance. Get enough to eat.

This is especially important if you have a history of eating disorders. For some eating-disorder survivors, adding new physical activity to their lives can trigger a resurgence of eating-disordered thinking because of old patterns of associating weight-loss dieting with exercise, or feeling that all physical activity *must* be associated with food restriction. Be gentle and kind with yourself if this begins to happen to you. Seek professional help if you think it would be useful to you. Talk to a trusted friend. Make plans to have meals with people who know your eating-disorder history and who will help you as you work to feed yourself normally and adequately. A good healthy body practice includes all aspects of your bodily and mental health, very much including your ability to feed yourself in ways that feel good and are sustainable.

Make Sure You're Eating a Variety of Foods That Provide All the Major Classes of Nutrients over the Course of Any Given Few Days

Our bodies need six major classes of nutrients to survive and be healthy: water, vitamins, minerals, fats, proteins, and carbohydrates. We also need dietary fiber to keep our gastrointestinal tracts functioning well. Calories, schmalories—this is the stuff you *really* have to pay attention to if you want to be able to be healthy, active, and full of mischief.

We can't get everything we need from one kind of food or one food group. Vitamin supplements are a useful security blanket and a good way to boost your nutrition, but they're not a great replacement for actual food. There's nothing wrong with taking vitamins, but for reasons we don't completely understand, the body uses the nutrients that are part of actual food more effectively than it can nutrients isolated in supplements.

You don't have to worry about getting every single type of nutrient in some mythical ideal balance at every meal. Your body, which evolved to make the most of whatever food could be scrounged up whenever it could be found, doesn't need to be micromanaged like that. Getting a good distribution and quantity of nutrients over the course of a couple of days will provide what your body needs to take care of the details. Given a reasonably balanced array of foods the rest of the time, you will not get scurvy, irrevocably ruin your metabolism, or otherwise hurt yourself if you happen to dine upon movie theater popcorn and Junior Mints once in a while. I happen to know this from personal experience and hands-on testing.

Pay Attention to How What You Eat Makes You Feel, and Adjust Accordingly

Different bodies thrive on different amounts and proportions of different kinds of foods. If you pay attention, your body will tell you loud and clear what it likes and what it doesn't. As Toronto nutritionist Michelle Allison puts it in her blog, The Fat Nutritionist, "Learning how food makes you feel, both immediately and a little way down the road, is a fundamental part of learning how to care for yourself. In my mind, food that makes you feel weird or off—no matter how good it tastes right now—isn't food you can unconditionally love."

Paying attention to how your food makes you feel begins with paying attention to when you're hungry and when you're full. Don't force yourself to eat when you aren't hungry. Don't refuse to eat when you are. It is totally appropriate to eat when you are hungry. That's why you *get* hungry. Hunger is not a moral issue. It is not your body's way of trying to trick you into doing something that is bad for you. It is just your body's subtle little way of saying that it needs supplies so it can do its job.

Paying attention to how your food makes you feel continues with noting how specific foods and food groups make you feel, both physically and mentally. Some people have strong physical reactions to particular eating patterns or types of foods. Others don't.

In figuring out what works best for you, you have the unparalleled luxury of being your own lab rat. Pay attention and you'll experience the results immediately. "Eating right" means eating what works best for your body and your brain, and the only person who can honestly evaluate that is *you*. (But do be honest, because you are also the only person you're going to hurt with dishonesty.)

Once you've figured it out, you need only do the best you can. Every time you have a meal or a snack, it's a chance to do your best to give yourself the things you specifically thrive on. Sometimes you can't. Sometimes you don't want to. Sometimes you do want to but you have a lot of difficulty in doing it. Sometimes you do it halfway. Sometimes you do it perfectly. Be patient. Keep practicing. The goal isn't to eat perfectly all the time (whatever that is, and as if you could!). The goal is to eat right for your own needs as much of the time as you can so you can feel your best.

Enjoy Your Food

Eating shouldn't be a punishment. If you're eating something you really don't like, there'd better be a damn good reason for you to inflict that kind of psychological and sensory nastiness on yourself. (Not offending your hosts at a dinner party may qualify.) There's a lot of physical good to be gotten out of physical pleasure. Eating good food, the best you can afford, prepared as well as you can manage it, improves your quality of life immeasurably, which helps keep you happy and healthy and sleek. Experiment! There are so many foods out there in the world, and most of them are pretty darn tasty. Just because you don't like zucchini doesn't mean you won't enjoy eggplant, butternut squash, or winter melon. Play with your food! Have fun mixing it up and exploring new things. The more foods you know you enjoy, the more enjoyable options you have.

When to Consult a Nutritionist

There are a few situations where people may want to seek out professional help in managing their eating in relation to their physical activity.

If you are an endurance athlete—a marathoner, triathlete, or the like—you may need to tailor your nutrition specifically to your needs as an athlete simply because you are pushing your body so hard for so long that normal eating just may not suffice. A qualified nutritionist can help you with that.

You may also want to talk to a nutritionist if you are diabetic. Many diabetics have predictable enough symptoms and patterns that they can manage their own nutrition and medication without help, even when they are changing their physical-activity levels. But this can be a complicated task for others, especially if you have diabetes that is brittle and hard to manage. Because diabetics need to be extra careful to eat and medicate to maintain a healthy blood glucose level around the clock, including during and after exercise, it can be helpful to consult a nutritionist with a diabetes specialty.

Nutrition and Physical Activity

Although there aren't many specific food rules that are really worth following, making sure you get good nutrition before, during, and after physical activity will improve your overall experience. You'll feel better, have fewer distractions, and have more of what your body needs to do all the things you want to do.

- **Don't exercise on a completely empty stomach.** Hunger pangs are distracting, annoying, and don't feel good. You want to be able to enjoy how it feels to move your body, not be constantly cranky because you're so hungry. If you haven't eaten anything in four or more hours, consider at least a small, nutrient-dense snack a half an hour before you hit the gym or go for that walk, paddle, ride, skateboard, or run. You want a small quantity of something that you will digest slowly and can give you energy over a long period so your blood sugar will remain reasonably stable. Some good options are some nuts or edamame, a glass of milk or soymilk, a sandwich, a hard-cooked egg, and crackers with some cheese or nut butter on them.

- **Avoid eating intensely sugary things as a preexercise snack.** They can set you up for a sugar high followed by a nasty crash when your exercising body burns right through all that sugar and you go *splat*. Some people are more strongly affected by these ups and downs than others, but they can be outright dangerous to people with a tendency to hypoglycemia. Even if you're not particularly affected by sugar surges, eating things that will produce less of a spike and less of a crash is still easier on your system.

- **Don't exercise on a very full stomach.** A big meal right before strenuous activity is a recipe for—*ulp!*—trouble. A mellow saunter around the neighborhood after dinner won't be a problem, but hopping right on your bike and heading over to that killer hill-climb route might end badly. Rather than end up feeling bloated, dyspeptic, or nauseated, give yourself an hour or two to digest a full meal before you start running around.

- **Don't worry about eating specific foods to try to produce particular kinds of athletic results.** Most people with moderately active lives don't worry about carb-loading, megadosing on protein to build muscle, or taking sports-related dietary supplements. Nor would it necessarily help them perform any better if they did: making nutritional materials available to the body does not automatically translate into the body using them in the specific ways you would like it to. If you're eating sufficient amounts of a reasonable variety of foods, your body will have what it needs to move, get stronger, build muscle, improve its reflexes, and all that good stuff. Improving your physical performance owes a hell of a lot more to consistent practice than it does to what you eat or what vitamins or supplements you take, in any case.

- **Drink plenty of water.** Staying hydrated is very important no matter what, and it's all the more important if you're sweating a lot. When we sweat, we lose both water and salts, which in sufficient quantity will affect your body's electrolyte balance. But don't be taken in by the electrolyte imbalance bogeyman: the body is typically completely capable of handling you getting hot and sweaty for a limited time without your electrolytes going into a tailspin, so long as you're eating and drinking adequately, including drinking enough during exercise or when you're sweating a lot. Get used to hitting that water bottle while you're moving your body! If you feel that you do want something to shore up your electrolytes just to be on the safe side, you can avoid the cost, the tooth decay, and the sugar roller coaster of high-sugar "sports drinks" by mixing up an easy, cheap homemade substitute that works every bit as well as a bottle of commercial sports drink. Simply mix up about a quarter teaspoon of salt and a tablespoon or two of sugar, plus a liberal squeeze of lemon or other citrus juice in a cup of water (multiply the proportions to make a larger quantity). A version of this is used by doctors around the world to restore electrolyte balance in people in danger of dying from the depletions of chronic vomiting or diarrhea. It dependably gets the job done under those circumstances, and will work fine for you too.

Sometimes people turn to sports drinks simply because they don't enjoy drinking plain water. If that's an issue for you, try the surprisingly delicious trick of infusing your H_2O with some sliced fruit (like lemon or orange), fresh herbs (like mint), or even sliced vegetables (like cucumber or tomato). Or try filling your water bottle with iced herbal tea. I particularly love zesty, fruity herbal teas for this because they are so good at cutting through the dry-mouth that sometimes happens when you're breathing hard. These are cheap, fresh, and tasty!

Getting Down (and Up Again)

One issue you won't see discussed in many other fitness books is the problem of getting up off the floor. No, I don't mean because you're so drunk you can't stand up once you've fallen over, either, and anyway that's not a *fitness* problem. I mean the problem of being unable, for one reason or another, to get back up on your feet again if you should happen to end up, intentionally or unintentionally, on the floor.

The prospect of being unable to get up off the floor is legitimately scary and humiliating. We want to be competent and capable human beings, and the idea that we could be incapable in this way can be deeply distressing.

There are many reasons that someone might be unable to get up off the floor. People of all different sizes and weights have problems with knees, wrists, and other joints. Regardless of size, some people do not have the functional fitness and muscular strength to lift their own body weight, which is what must be done if one is going to get up off a floor. Sometimes people's bodies are shaped in ways that make this more difficult, and sometimes being very heavy is also a contributing factor.

Do not be ashamed if you are afraid that you might not be able to get up off the floor. This is a reasonable fear! It is also reasonable to avoid getting down on the floor if you are afraid you might not be able to get back up again.

But do not let your fear or your shame keep you from working toward improving your functional fitness so that you do not have to be so scared. Getting down to the floor and back up again is something you can work toward. The physical strength and muscular skill it requires to get back up to your feet after being on the ground or the floor can, in most cases, be acquired or improved. Even if you never actually have to do it, it's good to know that you can.

Getting up off the ground requires strength in your legs, your arms, and your trunk. Here are some ways you can build strength in those parts of your body.

Legs

- Getting up from a chair uses a lot of the same muscles as getting up from the floor. Pick a chair and sit in it and then stand up. Sit back down and stand back up. Repeat ten times for a full set and work up to doing five sets. Once this feels relatively easy, cross your arms over your chest when you do it, increasing the difficulty and improving your trunk strength.

- Going up and down stairs also improves your leg strength. Not up to stairs? Try stepping up and down off of a curb or some other sturdy platform of reasonable size, like a step aerobics step (these are often stackable, so you can add height to the step as you are able).

- Stand in front of your couch or a soft chair with your back to it and with a kitchen chair (or other sturdy chair with a high back) in front of you. Hold on to the high-backed chair. Lift one foot up behind you, as if you were kicking someone behind you in line, and hook the top of that foot over the edge of the couch or soft chair. Press down as hard as you can with that foot. Hold for a count of five. Lower your leg and switch sides. Do each side five times for a complete set and work your way up to five sets.

- Walking, biking, water aerobics, swimming, water-walking, and many other activities build leg strength and are also good for general conditioning. Even if you are able to do only very short walks, such as walking around your home for a few minutes, it's better than no walking at all and will build strength if you stick with it.

Arms

- Pushing yourself up from the floor so you can get your legs under you takes a lot of the same muscles as when you push yourself up with your arms to get out of a chair. As in the exercise described above for the legs, work on rising and sitting and rising again from a chair, using your arms as much as possible to raise your body out of the chair. Ten repeats make a set. Work your way up to five sets.

- Using your body weight as resistance, you can also build arm strength by doing push-ups against a wall. Stand at arm's length from the wall with your palms flat against the wall at or just below shoulder height. Let yourself lean toward the wall, controlling your motion with your arms, until your forehead touches the wall. Then use your arms to push yourself back to a fully upright standing position. This exercise can also be done using other, lower surfaces, such as while hanging on to the back of a sofa.

- Put your palms together at chest level. Push one palm against the other as hard as you can. Then lace your fingers together and hold on tight while pulling your arms away from each other as hard as you can. Do this again: Flatten your hands and push! Then interlace your fingers and pull! Repeat this cycle ten times for one set. Work up to five sets.

- Lift a small but relatively heavy object, such as a bottle of water or a telephone book, in your hand, keeping your arm straight until you have raised your entire arm to shoulder height. Hold your arm there for a count of ten. Lower your arm again. Repeat five times, then do it on the other side. Work your way up to five sets.

INCENDIARY ACT #12

KNOW THAT YOU ARE THE AUTHORITY ON YOU

There are an awful lot of people who have an awful lot invested in keeping you convinced that you don't know what you're doing when it comes to your own body. The fashion industry depends utterly on convincing you that you don't know how to get dressed without someone else telling you what to wear. The diet industry would shrivel up and die if it weren't so good at making people believe that they don't know how to feed themselves properly and that they should not trust their bodies' own appetites and cues. The weight-loss industry could not do what it does without being able to convince you that the natural variability of body types is evidence that bodies, left to their own devices, will betray you every time by refusing to look the way you want them to. The food industry wants to mother-hen you with "healthy choices" and "smart ideas," insinuating that you're incapable of making any healthy decisions or having any intelligent thoughts about eating on your own.

The fitness industry is mostly no better. Everywhere you turn, there are people who will not wait to be asked for their advice before they tell you—on the assumption that you as a fat woman could not possibly know—how to move your body. You will find people who will lie to you with a straight face and tell you that their method, and only their method, will produce "real results," whatever it is they mean by that. You will encounter people who will condescend to you and treat you as though a fat body is proof positive that you are basically a blithering idiot. You will encounter people who insist that because you are fat, you are not a reliable witness about your own health or physical condition.

This book, although it is nominally a small slice of the fitness industry, does not endorse any of these ideas. The truth is that *you are the ultimate authority on you.* You live in your body 24/7. There is nobody who experiences it more personally, nobody who knows it in as many different moods and modes as you do, and nobody else who can tell you, immediately and without question, whether something feels good or bad, right or wrong, beneficial or harmful. You will be the first to know when your body practice is improving your quality of life, and you will be the first to know if you overdo something and end up sore or injured. You know when your eating patterns are making your body happy and when they're not; you know when you're feeling energetic and when you're feeling sluggish. You are completely capable of noticing and keeping track of your body's particular patterns and proclivities. You are totally and without question the person with the best possible authority to manage those patterns and take advantage of those proclivities.

You *are* the authority on you. You *do* know what you're doing when it comes to your own body. Take your time. Pay attention. Be honest. Be straight with yourself about what's working and what's not. In time you will learn how to trust that you really do have all the authority in the world when it comes to your own body, and what's more, there's every reason that you should.

Trunk

- Raising your trunk off the floor is not so different from raising your trunk off a bed. Sit on the edge of your bed with your legs hanging off the side. Lie down on your back. Using your arms to help you, sit up. Repeat this process five times for a set. Work up to five sets. When you can do five sets without trouble, do it without using your arms and work your way up to five sets that way.

- Another thing you can do from the bed to improve your trunk strength is to lie on your back, bend your arms and knees, point your elbows toward your knees, and then bring your elbows and knees as close together as you can, curling your torso. When you have gotten them as close as you can, hold that position for a count of five and then relax. Do it a total of five times for a complete set. Work up to five sets of five.

- Stand near a table or counter that is waist height or lower. Make sure the table or counter is clear. Lean forward and put your hands on the table, then slowly push your hands forward as if you were pushing something heavy off of the table or along the counter. Stretch as far as you can without losing your balance (and don't worry, the table/counter is there to help support you if you wobble), then straighten slowly back up. Repeat this ten times. Work up to three sets. When this becomes easy for you, pick a lower table or counter, or do it using a chair instead, and hold onto the chair seat, physically pushing the chair away from your body.

All of these exercises should be repeated several times a week. You might put together a routine where you pick one from each category every day, and rotate your way through them. As you repeat these exercises over time, you'll notice that they get easier, you can do them more quickly, and you find them less taxing. You should also notice that other things are getting easier and quicker: standing up from a chair, getting out of bed, picking things up off the floor, getting in and out of a car. These things are exactly the proof you're looking for that you are getting stronger. As you get stronger, you can begin to incorporate other physical activity into your life. Plus-size fitness instructor Kelly Bliss has some excellent fitness videos that can be done from a seated position; these are a fantastic tool when you are at this stage in increasing your functional fitness (see the Resource Guide).

Do not try going down to the floor and getting up from the floor again until you are pretty sure you can make it. As an interim measure, you might try moving from lying down on your back on a bed to getting up on all fours on a bed, then transferring to lying down on your back again. Being able to do this consistently and repeatedly is a fairly good indicator that you now possess the strength and coordination to get yourself up and down off the floor. The first time you try actually getting down and then up off the floor, though, you should make sure that you have, at the least, some sturdy furniture around to help with leverage both on the way down and on the way back up. For safety's sake, you should also make sure you have a friend nearby to hang out, give you a pep talk if desired, and to help you if you need help.

Getting up and down off the floor can be hard on your wrists, hands, and especially knees. Those with damage to these body parts should be particularly careful about practicing this maneuver. There really are no ways get from flat on the floor to up on your feet under your own power without involving some or all of these body parts. While it would be worth risking hurting yourself in order to get yourself back up on your pins in an emergency, it is not worth it otherwise. Let your common sense be your guide, don't take unnecessary chances, and work on making sure that you are strong enough to minimize the amount of wear and tear that movement, even getting up off the floor, will put on your already damaged joints.

In Case of Emergency

If somebody gets down on the ground and finds that he or she cannot get up under their own steam, don't panic. (Even if that somebody is you. If you can remember these instructions, you can tell people how to help you get up again.)

First, make sure that the person is not injured or in any kind of physical distress. If she or he is, call 911 for help because moving someone who is hurt or having some sort of health crisis can be risky, and you do not want to accidentally make things worse.

If the person is not already lying on his or her back or side, help position them and make sure they are comfortable and breathing easily.

Next, get a few other people to help you and collect some supplies. You will need a sturdy sheet such as a flannel sheet or woven blanket. (There are companies that sell purpose-built reinforced nylon lifting and transfer slings with handles for this purpose, but it is unlikely that you will have one at your disposal. Should you wish to acquire one, see the Resource Guide.)

Fold the sheet or blanket so that it is wider than the person you intend to lift, and tall enough to support the person from their shoulders to at least the mid-thigh.

There are two ways to deploy the sheet:

1. **If the person is lying on her or his back:** Lay the sheet or blanket out flat on the floor, above the person's head. Then help the person wriggle up onto the sheet/blanket until his or her whole body from shoulders to mid-thighs is over the blanket.

2. **If the person can roll easily:** Lay the sheet or blanket out flat on the floor next to the person, lined up so that when the person rolls onto it, she or he can roll so that the body from shoulders to just above the backs of the knees is over the blanket.

Once you have positioned the person on the blanket or sheet, have your helpers grab the edges of the fabric and begin by lifting the shoulders and back so that the person is in a sitting position. From there, you can lift the person, supporting the back and torso, so that the person can get his or her legs under his or her body. It is a good idea to have a spare person (or two) nearby at this point to help by taking the person's arms to help pull him or her up and forward and to steady the person as they get to their feet. Do not worry if you cannot do all this in one smooth motion. Take your time and be careful. It's better to take more time and be cautious than it is to drop someone. If you have serious doubts about your ability to do this safely, call in emergency professionals. Paramedics and firefighters are trained to move people of a range of sizes safely in emergencies.

Institutionalized Body Hatred and the Unapologetic Fat Girl

So let's say you're an unapologetic fat girl and you've been busting your abundant and delectable behind trying to get your body practice to a place that makes you happy. You've been working on getting your head to a place where it's happy about your body practice and your bountiful booty as well. Let's say you've been making all kinds of progress on the physical-activity front and on the self-acceptance front, and you're feeling pretty good. You're enjoying your body and what it can do for you, you're enjoying your movement and what it does for your body and your mind, and you're feeling good in your skin. It's pretty awesome, feeling physically empowered!

Then you walk into the gym and there's a sign: "Win Free Membership for a Year with Our Weight-Loss Challenge!" Suddenly, you don't feel so awesome about going in to swim that half mile you were planning on. When what your gym sees fit to reward people for is being thinner, not fitter, it's easy to feel like all the hard work you've put into being fitter is completely invisible and maybe worthless.

Or maybe you roll into work one day and there's someone in the break room who wants you to join your workplace-sponsored fitness and weight-loss group. It's hard to feel like your coworkers value you for who you are and what you contribute when they're so obviously passing judgment on your body while they pressure you to join in their competitive diet-and-exercise reindeer games.

Perhaps you show up to your new yoga class and you're all jazzed and then . . . every other word out of the instructor's mouth has something to do with weight loss or calories or something else along those lines. Oddly, you find it difficult to concentrate on your form and making sure you don't overextend that trick knee of yours because you're being distracted every six seconds by the instructor's weight-loss fetish. What's more, you're getting just a bit freaked out by what she must be thinking seeing you in that classroom, big as day.

What's the right-thinking unapologetic fat girl to do when confronted with such blatant institutionalized fat-phobia and body hatred? What can you do to combat these kinds of messages and this kind of treatment of unskinny bodies, including your own? How can you, at the very least, find ways not to be unduly affected by these messages and these dynamics when they surround you willy-nilly, so that you can protect your own mental health and equilibrium?

First, know what you're seeing when you see it. Strong, deeply ingrained prejudice against fat bodies and in favor of thin bodies is nearly everywhere in our culture. The fact that this bias exists does not make it correct, ethical, or moral. Your body is a valid and worthwhile body, no matter what size it is. Any message that tries to convince you otherwise is wrong. When you see or hear messages that try to tell you that the only way to have a worthwhile or acceptable body is to have a thinner body, to lose weight, or to look a certain thin way, know that this is prejudice talking, not reality.

Second, know that your body practice is your business and yours alone. Just because other people want to insist that they know better than you do what you should be doing with your body doesn't mean they actually do. It simply isn't anyone else's business what your body practice looks like, what your priorities for your body practice are, or how you choose to implement those priorities. One of the reasons people so often get away with telling other people how to conduct their body practice is that people have been taught that they are not competent to do it themselves. That's just not true. You are supremely competent to run your own body practice. You are the only person who ultimately *can* run your own body practice. . . . It's not like anyone else is going to haul your body off to the gym and exercise it for you while you sleep in, you know? You may as well own it!

Third, know that you can trust yourself about what is right for your body. No one knows more about what it's like to be inside your body than you do. No one knows more about what feels good and what feels bad, what works for you and what doesn't, than you. You are the one with all the feedback and all the access to every single sensation that tells you whether something makes your body happy. You are the decision maker because you are the expert on you.

Fourth, know that you can be healthy and happy in your body whether or not it is slender. Weight and size are only two of many, many things that make up our physical bodies and our physical experience. We do experience our bodies as having weight and as having size. But we also experience a lot of other things: whether we are energetic, strong, breathing easily and fully, whether our digestion is good, our muscles springy and elastic, our mood is stable and upbeat, and whether we seem to feel good in our skin. There are all kinds of ways in which we can feel good and feel happy in and about our bodies, and this can happen whether or not our bodies are slender. Being as healthy and as happy as you possibly can be in your body is not something that you have to be a certain weight to do! You can do it any time, at any size at all.

Fifth and last, know that you have a right to make yourself heard. When something offends you, irritates you, or makes you feel needlessly bad about yourself or your body practice, you have the right to say so. This does not mean that you are *obligated* to say something. There are countless instances of institutionalized and interpersonal body hatred in this world, and you could exhaust yourself trying to point them all out and still not really scratch the surface. If the situation is one that you can just roll your eyes at, one where it doesn't eat at you or raise your blood pressure, then leave it alone if you like. You don't have to be the Designated Fat Angel of Justice all the time.

But if a situation is making you angry or frustrated or if you find yourself unable to stop taking it personally, feeling attacked or belittled or dismissed, it is completely okay for you to say something. It is okay to go to the manager of your gym and explain exactly why you feel like your efforts to improve your *fitness* are rendered invisible when they hold a competition that only rewards losing weight. It is okay to go to your boss or your HR manager at work and say that you find it difficult to feel valued as a member of the work team when there is so much weight-loss rhetoric and competition in the workplace. It is more than acceptable to go to the yoga teacher after class and say, "I find your constant weight-loss talk very distracting; I am trying to concentrate on form and focus my breathing and it is hard for me to do that when I am being made to feel self-conscious and like I am not measuring up to an implied standard about what bodies are supposed to look like in this class." (And if it doesn't work, you can go over their heads.)

You may or may not be able to change things. People cling very hard to their prejudices about weight and size. But for your own sake as well as any change you may be able to effect, you can definitely make yourself heard.

Whether or not you choose to speak out or to engage in any form of activism around your own right to have access to fitness and movement that support *your* body and bodies like yours, ultimately the most important thing is that you just keep moving. The more you insist on the movement you want and need by simply doing it, the more you show the world that you, and other people like you, are every bit as entitled as anyone else to move and play and exist in the world in ways that delight you and improve your quality of life.

Epilogue: What Moves You

In the final analysis, your body practice is all about you. It is yours, utterly and completely, and the bottom line is nothing more or less than whether or not it works for you and gives you what you want and need. You don't have to settle for less than what makes you feel fierce! You don't have to settle for less than what makes you feel good in your skin! You have the right to move your body in any ways that move your soul, in any place you like, just because you want to. You have the right to make naysayers take responsibility for their bad attitudes and bad behavior, and simply cruise on, working your body practice like no one's watching for no other reason than because it makes you feel good.

You're worth it. Your body is a good body, and it is absolutely worth it too. You and your wonderful body are worth the work it takes, physical and mental, that helps you feel good and secure and strong in your skin. You deserve to feel strong and flexible and capable, full of energy and stamina and joie de vivre. Whatever your size, whatever your weight, however you might be shaped, you deserve to live in a body that feels as good and functions as well as it possibly can, and you are 100 percent entitled to every bit of positive, joyful movement and physicality that helps you get there.

At the beginning of this book I wrote about how movement gives your body back to you, and this is precisely what I meant. Living out loud, living fully and freely in your full-figured self, is a full-contact sport . . . and in a world that wants to tell you that you're not entitled to that kind of good life because your body doesn't fit some arbitrary set of standards, it may just be the ultimate incendiary act.

Resource Guide

This resource guide is by no means comprehensive. It is intended to point the reader toward a select group of carefully chosen, hand-picked favorite resources and to alert you to the existence of products, services, and information you may not otherwise encounter. There are, of course, hundreds of thousands of fitness resources that may appeal to the right-thinking unapologetic fat girl. I have tried to err on the side of choosing those with a resolutely body-accepting, diversity-conscious slant. It is highly likely that you have your own favorites that are not included in this list; I apologize that I cannot possibly include them all.

Every effort has been made to ensure that the information in this resource guide is up to date and accurate. Inevitably, by the time you read this, some of it will no longer be. Consult the oracle of the Internet; much may be revealed.

Required Reading

These books are my personal short list of the best out there on the subject of weight, fitness, activity, and health. You owe it to yourself to add these to your library and your knowledge base.

Bacon, Linda. *Health At Every Size: The Surprising Truth About Your Weight.* Dallas, TX: BenBella Books, 2010.

Bliss, Kelly. *Don't Weight: Eat Healthy and Get Moving Now.* West Conshohocken, PA: Infinity Publishing, 2002.

Chastain, Ragen. *Fat: The Owner's Manual*. Austin, TX: Sized for Success Multimedia, 2012.

DePatie, Jeannette. *The Fat Chick Works Out: Fitness That's Fun and Feasible for Folks of All Ages, Sizes, Shapes, and Abilities*. Los Angeles, CA: Real Big Publishing, 2011.

Lyons, Pat, and Debby Burgard. *Great Shape: The First Fitness Guide for Large Women*. Boulder, CO: Bull Publishing Co., 1990.

Rice, Rochelle. *Real Fitness for Real Women: A Unique Workout Program for the Plus-Size Woman*. New York: Grand Central Publishing, 2001.

Wann, Marilyn. *Fat!So?: Because You Don't Have to Apologize for Your Size*. Berkeley, CA: Ten Speed Press, 1998.

Additional Reading

These books and blogs represent a selection of good resources having to do specifically with fitness, weight, activity, and health. There are many others out there that you may also wish to look into, but these are consistently good and useful and devoid of body shaming.

Anderson, Bob. *Stretching*. Bolinas, CA: Shelter Publications, 2010.

Bliss, Kelly. *Plus Size Yellow Pages* (website). www.plussizeyellowpages.com. (Especially good are the sections on sportswear, swimwear, and plus-size fitness.)

Chastain, Ragen. *Dances with Fat* (blog). http://danceswithfat.wordpress.com.

Kerr, Meera. *Big Yoga: A Simple Guide for Bigger Bodies*. Garden City Park, NY: Square One Publishers, 2010.

National Institutes of Health. *Active At Any Size* (downloadable PDF). http://win.niddk.nih.gov/publications/active.htm

Poretsky, Golda. *Body Love Wellness* (blog). www.bodylovewellness.com/blog.

Robison, Jon. *10 Things You Can Do Right Now To Ease Concerns About Your Weight & Improve Your Health*. (downloadable PDF). http://jonrobison.net/wp-content/uploads/2010/12/10_things_robison2.pdf.

Schiraldi, Glenn. *The Post-Traumatic Stress Disorder Sourcebook: A Guide to Healing, Recovery, and Growth.* New York: McGraw-Hill, 2000.

Williams, Jayne. *Shape Up with the Slow Fat Triathlete: 50 Ways to Kick Butt on the Field, in the Pool, or at the Gym—No Matter What Your Size and Shape.* Boston, MA: Da Capo Press Lifelong Books, 2008.

Size-Accepting Exercise Instruction

The following titles are DVDs. Some of these instructors also teach privately or in group settings, and many have their own websites. Search for them online by name to find out more about a particular instructor or to locate these DVDs. Be sure to look at Phat Moves (http://phatmoves.com), a clearinghouse for size-accepting fitness videos, including many listed below, and other helpful items.

Bliss, Kelly. *Standing Aerobics* and *Sitting Aerobics.*

Bliss, Kelly. *SuperFit: Sitting Aerobics Workout.*

DePatie, Jeanette. *The Fat Chick Works Out.* Los Angeles, CA: Real Big Publishing, 2006.

Garcia, Megan. *MegaYoga.* New York: Simba Productions, 2005, 2011.

Kerr, Meera. *Big Yoga Flex-Ability.* Big Yoga Studios, 2010.

Lentz, Abby. *HeavyWeight Yoga 1 and 2.* Austin, TX: HeartFelt Yoga, 2007.

Mack, Debby. *Debby Mack's Fitness 101, Debby Mack's PlusSize Workouts.* Warren, OH: Clear Choice Creative Corp., 2010.

Rice, Rochelle. *Empowering Women Through Movement.* New York: Kipany Productions Limited, 2008.

Robinson, Lynne. *Look Great Feel Great: Plus-Size Pilates.* Richardson, TX: Well Go USA Entertainment, 2008.

Stolove, Jodi. *Chairdancing.* (See also numerous other titles in this series.) Del Mar, CA: Chair Dancing International, 2004.

Self-Training Programs

Clark, Josh. *The Couch-to-5K Running Program.* www.coolrunning.com/engine/2/2_3/181.shtml.

This is a self-led training program for running that aims to get the user to the point where he or she can run 5K (or thirty minutes) in eight weeks. This may not be realistic for everyone. However, each week's workouts are carefully graduated and calibrated to build strength and stamina, and you can repeat a week as often as you need to until you are ready to move on. This is a perfect example of how you can use interval training over time to meet a dramatic fitness goal.

Nichols, Nicole. *Walking Workouts with Intervals.* www.sparkpeople.com/resource/fitness_articles.asp?id=1221.

There are numerous versions of this kind of walking workout available online. This page from Sparkpeople.com has three interval-training walking workouts, graded by intensity. For those wanting examples of how to alternate periods of more and less intense activity in their workouts, this is a good illustration, useful and sensible.

Speirs, Steve. *Two Hundred Sit-Ups.* www.twohundredsitups.com.

This is a self-led training program that uses interval-training principles to build stamina and capacity for this important back, core, and abdominal strength exercise. If you are not a fan of traditional sit-ups, you can use the same program to do crunches, exercise-ball sit-ups, and so on. Or modify it by using whatever core exercise you like best and benefit from the most. Feel free to repeat a week as often as you like before moving on to the next week.

Plus-Size Exercise Clothing and Sports Bras

A Big Attitude (http://abigattitude.com)

Plus-size quality sportswear for women with an extensive selection of products that run to 6X. Their bike shorts and capris have a deeply devoted following.

Champion (www.championusa.com)

Many products in sizes to 4X, made by a traditional sportswear manufacturer. Their sports bras are decent and reasonably priced. Look for their "Double Dry" technical fabric items.

Danskin (www.danskin.com)

Dancewear, leotards, tights, and other workout wear in sizes to 4X. Some people feel that the sizes run small. If you fit their sizes, they're a good source for basics that wear reasonably well.

Enell (http://enell.com)

The cult-favorite sports bra for well-endowed women. They offer off-the-rack sizes to approximately a 50DD, and custom sizing available for an additional setup charge.

Junonia (www.junonia.com)

The mothership of high-end plus-size sportswear and active-lifestyle fashion. The goods are expensive but also tend to be extremely high quality and to wear extremely well, with well-chosen fabrics. They have extremely good (though pricey) water-exercise clothing, including rash guards, shorts, and aquatards of various levels of coverage.

Just My Size (www.justmysize.com)

An attractive price point for activewear and sports bras of reasonable quality in sizes that in many items run to 5X and in bras to 58J. Chlorine-resistant swimsuits at competitive prices are something to watch for here.

Liquid Fit Wetsuits (http://liquidfit.com)

Custom-made wetsuits, constructed to your precise measurements. No, they're not cheap, but they will fit your specific body, as their website copy says, "like it was poured on you."

Love Your Peaches (www.loveyourpeaches.com)

Catsuits, leotards, gorgeous bathing suits, and a line of very well-made jersey activewear items that can be worn in and out of the gym. They have sizes to 6X and lovely fabrics.

Oddessy Martial Arts Supply (http://oddessy.com)

Specialists in large-size martial arts uniforms with sizes to fit up to a forty-two-inch thigh and seventy-two-inch waist. Call them for assistance.

River's Edge Dancewear (www.riversedgedancewear.com)

Features a good selection of the highly regarded Bal Togs plus-size dance-wear line, including leotards, unitards, skirts, and beyond. Be aware that dancewear sizing runs significantly smaller than fashion-industry sizing, so refer to the measurement charts.

ShimmySista (http://shimmysista.com)

Belly dance gear to size 3X. They have many gorgeous items that could be worn anywhere, not just for dance.

Helpful Tools, Gadgets, Products, and References

Anti–Chub-Rub Lubricants

There are a variety of these lubricants. They are typically sold as "anti-chafe" solutions for runners, but you don't have to be a runner to benefit from them; you just have to have thighs that touch when you move around. Bodyglide (http://bodyglide.com) is perhaps the most popular brand, though there are others out there.

Double-Thickness Yoga Mats

These are useful for all kinds of floor exercises. There are several manu-facturers that make them, and you can find them at many sporting goods stores. Occasionally, you will also see yoga mats that are wider than average. Double-thickness mats are not necessarily any wider but do provide extra cushioning that can be useful.

Extra-Wide Bicycle Seats

These can make cycling more comfortable and sustainable. There are several manufacturers that make these. A good cycling shop should be able to help you find one if they don't stock them already. Not all big riders need a wider seat. The seat of your bike should support your sit bones and not a whole lot more: too wide a seat can lead to discomfort and chafing due to pressure being exerted on the groin area.

The Fat-Friendly Health Professionals List

(www.cat-and-dragon.com/stef/Fat/ffp.html)

This is a user-curated list of health care professionals around the world who are known to be size-accepting or fat-friendly—an excellent place to look for a new doctor.

Heavy-Duty Bicycles and Tricycles (www.supersizedcycles.com)

These are built very sturdily and can support far heavier riders than average road bikes. The drawback to these bikes is that they are themselves quite heavy. Worksman, Supersized Cycles, and New Leaf are three companies that build heavy-duty bicycles that can handle riders up to 550 pounds. See their website for details. There are many other bike and trike brands that work well for big riders, including Electra and even some models of the old standby, Schwinn.

Kneesavers (http://kneesavers.net)

These are custom pedal extenders for bicycles and stationary bicycles that extend the pedal further out to the side, allowing for a more natural motion when pedaling. They fit between the crank arm and the pedal.

Super Sling

This is a purpose-built, heavy-duty fabric lifting sling with integral handles that is specifically designed to enable helpers to lift a very large person from the floor to their feet. For gyms and fitness professionals who work with fat clients, it's definitely something to consider having on hand in case of emergency. Available from More of Me to Love (http://store.moreofmetolove.com).

Treadmill Desk

This is an idea developed by Dr. John Levine of the Mayo Clinic. The notion is that a standing desk built over a treadmill will allow the user to walk very slowly in place (at usually around one mile per hour) while working. For low-impact movement that fits in very well with your workday—or your at-home Internet time, for instance—this is a wonderful idea and a great option that can work well even for people with low functional fitness. If you can walk, you can walk at a treadmill desk. There are several websites with information on how to build your own treadmill desk inexpensively (used treadmills are easy to find for cheap!), such as www.treadmill-desk.com. Or, if you're feeling flush, there are commercial treadmill desks that are designed and manufactured for the purpose.

About the Author

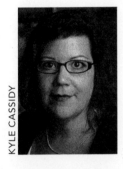

KYLE CASSIDY

HANNE BLANK spends her time thinking, learning, writing, and speaking at the crossroads of bodies, self, and culture. Joyfully spanning the town-gown divide as well as the mind-body split, her books include the histories *Straight: The Surprisingly Short History of Heterosexuality* (Beacon Press, 2012) and *Virgin: The Untouched History* (Bloomsbury, 2007), the cult classic sex and body-acceptance book *Big Big Love: A Sex and Relationships Guide for People of Size (and Those Who Love Them)* (Celestial Arts, 2011), and numerous others.

Hanne's work has been featured in periodicals ranging from *Penthouse* to *Bitch: Feminist Response to Pop Culture*, and in anthologies ranging from *Embodied Resistance: Challenging the Norms, Breaking the Rules* (Vanderbilt University Press, 2011) to *Fucking Daphne: Mostly True Stories and Fictions* (Seal Press, 2008) to *Yes Means Yes! Visions of Female Sexual Power and a World Without Rape* (Seal Press, 2008).

A former scholar of the Institute for Teaching and Research on Women at Towson University, Hanne has taught in various capacities on campuses including Brandeis and Tufts. She is also a popular speaker and guest lecturer, with appearances ranging from Harvard University to the inaugural Femme Conference and on topics from the history of the hymen to sex tips for people of all sizes.

Hanne lives in a vast old Victorian house in central Massachusetts but travels frequently to speak, teach, and perform. She is a rambling fat walker, a slow-and-steady fat bicyclist, a happy fat swimmer, and a regular high-reps-low-weights fat weightlifter who sometimes cheats on her old faithful, the elliptical trainer, with her new flame, the arc trainer. Find her online at www.hanneblank.com.

Index

C

Chafing, 166–67, 172–73, 202
Change
    of appearance, desires for, 23–24, 52–53
    inevitability of, 152
    reactions to, 152–54, 159–61
    types of, 153–54
    wanted vs. unwanted, 155–56, 158
Chub rub. *See* Chafing
Chunky Dunk, 66–67
Classes
    choosing, 78–79, 109
    fat-friendly, 65
    starting, 80
Clothing
    for belly flop, 128
    bras, 127–28, 200–201
    choosing, 122–25
    skinny jeans, 30
    skirts, 173
    sources of, 200–202
    swimsuits, 118
Community centers, 64–65
Comparisons, giving up, 150
Competitiveness, 77
Compliments, 55–57
Concern trolling, 57–58, 60
Console game–based fitness options, 82–83
Cool-down period, 141–42
Coordination
    activities for, 93
    definition of, 91
Cycling, 172, 202, 203

D

Dance
    clothing for, 201–2
    video games for, 83
Dehydration, 183–84

Diabetes, 181
Digestive system, 15
Dizziness, 165
Doctors
    avoiding scale at, 176
    blaming behaviors by, 176
    looking for, 202
    preparing for visits to, 174–75
    redirecting conversations with, 175
    with sports medicine subspecialty, 177
DOMS (delayed onset muscle soreness), 167–68
DVDs, 81–82, 199

E

Eating disorders, 179
80 percent rule, 42, 138–41, 160
Electrolyte balance, 183
Elliptical trainers, 172
Emergencies, 164–65, 189–90
Endorphins, 15
Exercise
    benefits of, 2–3, 5, 12–13, 14–16
    boredom and, 37–39
    connotations for, 27
    difficulty of, 6
    expectations for, 18, 149–52
    feedback on, 29–35
    group, 78–80
    at home, 80–83
    importance of, 2–3, 5
    instructional DVDs for, 81–82, 199
    misconceptions about, 52–53
    motivation and, 10–11, 18, 41, 130–33
    movement modification and, 146–47
    outdoors vs. indoors, 73–75
    partnerships, 76–78

phases of relationship to, 133–38
psychological boundaries
    surrounding, 18, 51–53
resuming, after break, 42–43
solo, 75–76
starting program of, 143–44
stealth, 70–73
substituting other words for,
    27–28
time of day for, 172, 182
See also Body practice; Workouts;
    individual exercises
Exercise bikes, 172
Expectations, managing, 18, 52–53,
    149–52

F

Fat
    -friendly environments, 64–67,
        110–11
    health and, 28–29
    use of word, 13
Fat-phobia
    institutionalized, 191–94
    prevalence of, 19–20
    See also Harassment
Fear, 18, 21, 58–59
Feedback, getting, 29–35
Feet
    painful, 168–69
    swollen, 172
Feldenkrais Method, 93
Fingers, swollen, 171
Fitness equipment
    comfort and ergonomics issues
        with, 103, 120–22
    at gyms, 103, 107–8
    shopping for, 122
    weight limits for, 119–20
Fitness industry, 87, 187
Flailing proudly, 84

Flexibility
    activities for, 93
    definition of, 91
Floor, getting up off, 184–86, 188–90
Food
    as energy source, 178
    enjoying, 181
    paying attention to impact of, on
        body, 180–81
    variety of, 179–80
    See also Eating disorders
Footwear, 125–27
Form, proper, 146–47
Functional fitness
    approaches to, 92–94
    components of, 91
    definition of, 90
    importance of, 90
Fungal infections, 173

G

Guilt, 21, 42
Gym bag, packing, 112–13
Gyms
    accessibility of, 102–3,
        105, 106
    child care at, 106
    choosing, 104, 105–11
    classes at, 109
    community centers vs., 64–65
    cost of, 109–10
    equipment and facilities at,
        103, 107–8
    fat-friendly, 110–11
    hours of, 106
    location of, 106
    locker rooms at, 111–14
    showers at, 114–15
    social factors for, 106–7
    specialized, 65, 105
    trying out, 105

H

HAES (Health At Every Size)
    approach, 28–29, 79
Harassment
    dealing with, 48–49, 60–62
    effects of, 46–47
    internalizing, 50–51, 58–59
    See also Advice, unsolicited;
        Compliments; Concern trolling;
        Fat-phobia
Headaches, 165
Health care professionals. *See* Doctors;
    Medical exercise specialists;
    Physical therapists
Heart attack, symptoms of, 164–65
Heart rate
    as feedback method, 31–32
    maximum, 31
    racing, 165
    resting, 32
    target range for, 31
Home, exercising at, 80–83
Hunger, 180, 182
Hydration, 183–84

I

Immune system, 14
Indoor vs. outdoor environments,
    73–75
Injuries, 165–71
Interval training, 142

J

Joints
    menstruation and, 173
    pain in, 171
Jones, Dhani, 84
Journaling, 34

K

Kinect, 82–83

L

Legs
    building strength in, 185
    chafing between, 166–67,
        172–73, 202
    swollen, 172
Lentz, Abby, 42
Levine, John, 203
Locker rooms, 111–14
Long-Haul Slump, 130–33
Lubricants, anti-chafing, 172–73, 202

M

Marla, Glenn, 7
Martial arts
    meditation and, 38
    uniforms for, 202
Medical exercise specialists, 177
Meditation, exercise as, 38,
    135–36
Menstruation, 173
Motivation, 10–11, 18, 41,
    130–33
Movement modification, 146–47
Muscle soreness, 167–68

N

Nintendo Wii, 82–83
Nutrition, 178–84
Nutritionists, 181

O

Outdoor vs. indoor environments,
    73–75
Overload, principle of, 138

P

Pain
    intense, 164
    joint, 171
    muscle soreness, 167–68
    plantar fascitis, 168–69
    shin splints, 168
    strains and sprains, 169–70
    stress fractures, 170–71
Partnerships, 76–78
Perfectionism, 51–52
Personal bests, 77
Personal trainers
    alternatives to, 176–77
    benefits of having, 86
    certification of, 87
    interviewing, 87–90
    limitations of, 87
Physical therapists, 177
Physicians. *See* Doctors
Pilates, 199
Plantar fascitis, 168–69
Practice, role of, 19–21
Prejudice. *See* Fat-phobia;
        Harassment

R

Record keeping, 32–35
Rehabilitative exercise specialists, 177
Resting heart rate, 32
Rice, Rochelle, 79
RICE (rest, ice, compression,
        elevation) protocol, 170
Rockport Walking Test, 33
Routine, establishing, 72–73
Running
    self-training program
        for, 200
    shoes for, 126

S

Scales
    avoiding, at doctors' offices, 176
    limitations of, 29–30
    Wii Fit balance board as, 82
Self-training programs, 200
Shin splints, 168
Shoes, 125–27
Showers, 114–15
Sit-ups, 200
Size
    acceptance, 28–29, 64–67, 110–11
    changes in, 159–61
Skeletal concerns, 170–71
Skinny jeans, as feedback method, 30
Skin problems, 165–67
Skirts, 173
Sleep, 14, 172
Slings, 190, 203
Solo exercise, 75–76
Soreness, 167–68
Spanx, 128
Special populations, fitness classes
        for, 65
Sports
    individual, 85–86
    team, 85–86
Sports bras, 127–28, 200, 201
Sports drinks, 183
Sports medicine physicians, 177
Sprains, 169–70
Stair climbers, 172
Stamina
    activities for, 93
    definition of, 91
Stealth exercise, 70–73
Strains, 169–70
Strength
    activities for, 93
    building, 184–86, 188–89
    definition of, 91

Stress fractures, 170–71
Stress reduction, 14
Stretching, 141
Stroke, symptoms of, 164–65
Sugar, 182
Supplements, 179
Swimming, 117–19, 172
Swimsuits, 118

T

Teachable moments, 61–62
Team sports, 85–86
Treadmills
    desks with, 203–4
    80 percent rule applied to, 139
Tricycles, 203
Trunk, building strength in, 188

U

Ultimate authority, you as, 41, 157,
    186–87, 192, 195

V

Varicose veins, 172
Vertigo, 165
Video games, 82–83
Visual disturbances, 165
Vitamin supplements, 179
VO$_2$max, 30–31

W

Walking
    self-training program for, 200
    shoes for, 126
    speed of, 32–33
Warm-up period, 141
Warning signs, 164–65
Water, importance of, 183–84
Water exercise, 117–19, 127
Weight
    changes in, 159–61
    loss as goal, 90
    See also Scales
Wetsuits, 201
Wii, 82–83
Workouts
    sample, 143–46
    structuring, 141–43

X

Xbox Kinect, 82–83

Y

Yoga
    instructional DVDs for, 199
    mats, 202
    movement modification and, 147

More Incendiary Advice
from Hanne Blank

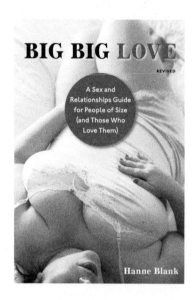

BIG BIG LOVE

A Sex and Relationships Guide for People of Size
(and Those Who Love Them)

REVISED

Paperback ISBN: 978-1-58761-085-1
E-book ISBN: 978-1-58761-371-5

Available from Ten Speed Press wherever books are sold.
www.tenspeed.com